Raving
Patients®

A System of Practical, Research-based Techniques
for Improving Healthcare Provider/Patient
Communication and Outcomes

Brenton B. Koch, MD, FACS

Author of

50 Questions (You MUST Ask!) Before You Have Plastic Surgery

Southfork Publishing
Brenton Koch, MD, FACS
4855 Mills Civic Parkway, Suite 100
West Des Moines, IA 50265
(515) 277-5555
Koch@kochmd.com

Printed in the United States of America
First Printing, 2013

ISBN-13: 9781481250856

ISBN-10: 148125085X

Cover design by Estela Jia Ceyril A. Redulla

Table of Contents

For the tiny, bald girl in the Minnie Mouse hospital gown who taught me everything I need to know about compassion in medicine.

People pay the doctor for his trouble;
for his kindness they still remain in his debt.

— Seneca

Introduction

*And each in the cell of himself is almost
convinced of his freedom.*

—W. H. Auden

Many of us can point to one day that changed the trajectory of our lives forever, and I am no exception. My big day — my Day of No Return, as I like to call it — came during my third year of head and neck surgery residency at the University of Iowa, one of the largest hospitals in the nation. The head and neck surgery residency there is among the best in the world. It is an overwhelmingly busy and pressure-packed environment, very demanding of the people who work within it. During my time there, we dealt day in, day out with a steady parade of cancer patients and skull-base surgery patients one after the other. I was on a large team of residents and attending physicians, and I was taking call in-house (meaning overnight call) every third night in addition to making daily rounds. I was at the hospital far more than I was home. This was in the era before mandatory eighty-hour-week limits were instituted. I saw my dog more often than I saw my wife, who was a second-year resident in pediatrics. Our marriage was crumbling as a result.

One cold, midwinter day, I was privileged to be involved in a surgical procedure that ran for eighteen hours on an unfortunate gentleman who had cancer of the midface and palate and the floor of his left orbit. We removed half of his palate and a sizeable portion of his left facial skin. We enucleated his left eye. A portion of his skull base on the left was removed in order to clear the cancer, and we reconstructed this skull-base area with a piece of his scapula via free-tissue transfer. We used the overlying skin accompanying the bone harvested from his upper back to rebuild the lining of his mouth and his palate, then we took a portion of his forearm skin to rebuild that which we took away over the face, and to fill in the orbit.

After the surgery it was my responsibility to transport him into the surgical intensive care unit, get orders written, and make sure the patient was stable postoperatively. It was 3:00 a.m. by the time I finished this. I had to start rounds two hours later, so there was no sense in driving home. I settled in the call room, but I couldn't sleep because the on-call resident kept me awake with his necessary coming and going.

I showered two hours later and started my rounds for the morning, but they were interrupted by an ICU nurse who called to tell me the patient from the night before was having a problem. There was no pulse in the flap in the palate, meaning the reconstructive piece in the mouth wasn't getting blood supply. Bad news. I went up and confirmed that was the case. We—the same team that had done the previous surgery—took the patient back to the operating room for another six hours to reconnect the blood supply. Then I was on call that night, which meant beginning at 5:00 p.m., my beeper was going to start its notices of patient needs and nurse requests. Consults on the floor and patient problems would become *my* responsibility for the rest of the night, and the emergency department would welcome a steady stream of facial injuries.

Around seven o'clock that evening, I was up on one of the inpatient floors sitting with my head in my hands, staring at the floor. A nurse asked me what was wrong.

"I'm tired. I don't want to do this anymore," I said.

I was completely burnt out and exhausted. I hadn't slept in forty hours. But there would be no rest for me still, because at that moment I was called to the emergency room to see yet another patient. As I waited to get on the elevator, I found myself behind a woman who was struggling with an IV pole and its bulky pump attachment. One of the five little wheels on the pole—which had a bag of IV solution swinging precariously from the top of it—was stuck in the gap between the floor and the elevator. The woman was dressed in well-worn jeans and an old T-shirt, and her disheveled hair was pulled back in a low ponytail. She continued to try to force the wheels to roll over the gap, and as I stood there waiting for her to get out of my way I got increasingly impatient. Couldn't she see I was in a hurry?

In a huff I growled, "Come on! Just pick it up!" I reached around her, picked up the pole, moved it forward, and plunked it down, clearing the way for me to board the elevator.

The woman turned to face me.

"You don't have to be *that* way," she said.

"Yes, I do have to be that way. I have to get to the emergency room," I replied with all of the smug superiority to which I was unentitled as a third-year resident.

I stepped farther into the elevator and there, standing in the corner behind this woman's legs, was a little girl, probably four years old, wearing a baggy, little hospital gown covered with a Minnie Mouse print. The line from the same IV pole ran into her tiny, bruised arm. She was bald—obviously a cancer patient. The little girl looked up at me. I looked away, punched the number for my floor, and stared at the ceiling for the remainder of my ride.

As the evening wore on and the unrelenting demands on my body and mind continued, I got more frustrated and irritable by the minute. I hated this place...these people...this work. I had left the emergency room, made several trips across the massive hospital to complete various requests, and was on my way back up to the floor when I went around a corner and there, near the same elevator as before, were the mom and the little girl. They were walking at a snail's pace away from me, about twenty feet ahead. Through the opening in the back of the child's hospital gown, I could see her little underpants drooping off her emaciated body. I could see her pencil-thin legs wobbling with every tiny step she took.

Suddenly she stopped walking and eased herself down to sit on one of the legs of the IV pole. Her mom halted, turned back, and asked, "Honey, what are you doing?"

And the little girl looked up at her mom and said: "I'm tired. I don't want to do this anymore."

In that moment I felt as if a ton of bricks had landed on me. That poor, little girl said exactly the same words I had said to the nurse earlier that night but for completely different reasons — and hers were so much more important and valid than mine.

I walked quickly around the corner before the mother and child could see me. Blinded by shame-filled tears, I stumbled through the exit doors and out into the atrium, out into the frigid Iowa night. I slumped onto a bench, buried my head in my hands, and sobbed like a child.

That was when everything changed for me. I realized the way I was looking at my profession was dead wrong. I had been taking everything for granted. And, even worse, I had been a self-centered ass about it.

In that moment I started to take myself a lot less seriously and take my work more seriously. It is an amazing gift to be in a position to help a little cancer patient and her mother, who never deserved my snide comment on the elevator.[1] I started to communicate with my patients differently, meaning I worked hard to understand them in a way I hadn't before. I began focusing more on them and less on myself. I began trying hard to convey what I meant in a new and more compassionate way — just as I know all of us can if we're doing this work for the right reasons. The result was that my career changed for the better…and so did every other aspect of my life.

The goal of this book is to revolutionize healthcare — one patient at a time — by instructing doctors, nurses, physician assistants, nurse practitioners, and other ancillary healthcare professionals in the fine art of providing exemplary customer service. There are many reasons why this is an important goal, and

---

1 I never apologized to her mom because I was just too embarrassed. I regret that to this day.

thanks to the hard lesson I learned from little Sarah and her mom so many years ago, I am determined to do my part to achieve it.

I suspect I don't need to tell you the level of respect for the healthcare industry and healthcare providers has taken a sharp nosedive, and it's not going to be recovered by continuing on our present course. I am old enough to remember the proverbial town doctors who were the pillars of their communities. In addition to running thriving medical practices, these people were on the school board and the arts council. They coached Little League, and they were active in the civic clubs that worked to make life better for everyone in the area. They were the guy or gal next door with all the answers. They were the people you could trust with your life, with your kids' lives. You knew them well, and they knew you. You could count on them to be there 24/7.

Those days are gone. Now the arts council meeting degenerates into an argument over Obamacare. A visit to someone's home becomes a risk should a medical emergency occur and you are viewed as not responding appropriately. I have a medical colleague who coached his daughter's pee wee soccer team and was threatened with a lawsuit when one of the little players sustained a cut on the forehead during an innocent practice drill. Her parents told him, "You're a doctor. You should know better!" Apparently accidents do not happen when you're a doctor.

The same frustrations hold true for the patient. Now if little Jenny is sick, you take her to the walk-in clinic, fork over your co-pay, and settle in for a lengthy wait in a lobby filled with ten other rashy, sneezy kids and magazines that were current during the Reagan administration. When you finally get to see a doctor (who is probably someone you've never met before), he bursts into the room behind schedule and distracted. He's tired because he's pressured to see more patients in less time, and he's seen a dozen kids already this morning. He spends more time typing notes on his iPad than he does interacting with you and Jenny. He is careful not to suggest any particular course of treatment for your child but instead provides a veritable buffet of therapeutic options and tells you to pick one. He doesn't want to commit to anything because that would make him more likely to be sued should anything unpredicted occur.

So essentially you and Jenny are no better off than when you walked into the doctor's office, but now you're even more frustrated, even more cranky, and a few bucks poorer to boot. And your level of respect for the healthcare industry just tumbled downward a few more degrees.

It's almost as if our profession is trying to speed up the powerboat while simultaneously dragging an anchor behind us. We healthcare providers are spending less and less time with our patients, yet we expect more and more pay. Imagine if your house painter were to spend less time painting each day but still demanded to be paid the same amount. It doesn't work that way in the house painting business. To think that it ought to work that way for us as healthcare providers is simply a misguided expectation.

Now, I'm not saying this downward spiral is entirely the fault of individual doctors and nurses. I recognize that our current system is a pressure cooker from the top down. This pressure cooker is causing increased frustration and compounded uncertainty about what the future holds, particularly with the political changes on the horizon. Regulations are expanding. Malpractice premiums and awards continue to skyrocket. Healthcare professionals are forced to log more paperwork, make more computer entries, and cram more patient visits into each day because more patient visits mean more money coming into the medical machine. Patients don't seem to be people anymore. They are codes that need to be generated. Mrs. Smith isn't a woman; she's Code 99242. Remember to check the box beside the number. You do not want another audit by accounts receivable, do you?

Medicine is about more than just treating sick people. It's also about helping people feel better about themselves.

The healthcare system seems to have forgotten that we are an industry of service providers. We are in the customer service business. We are in the sales business. Our job is to sell an uninformed consumer health and wellness—to sell them on the notion that they can take an active role in overcoming many of the things that ail them. I'm not saying you can cure cancer by believing that, but I am saying there are a growing number of diagnoses that are self-generated. Smoking, alcoholism, drug abuse, and morbid obesity can be controlled from the patient side, and we can help people do that—but only if we are providing exemplary customer service. By maximizing our time, listening attentively to our patients, and making appropriate sales pitches to them, we can convince them they have the power to make themselves better—and healthy again.

When we engage in positively framed, sincere dialogues with our patients, we will be more effective. Our message will resonate and become imprinted on their brains. They'll be more likely to remember our advice and instructions. They'll be more likely to have a positive outcome.

But not if they have to wait an hour or more in a crowded lobby after receiving a curt greeting from the person at the reception desk. Not if they encounter three different people during their visit who never smile at them or look them in the eye. Not if the doctor breezes in and spends a grand total of three minutes in the room with her hand on the doorknob the entire time.

Think about it this way: Imagine if a neighbor came to your home and rang your doorbell. You would probably open the door, greet her with a warm smile, welcome her in, and do everything in your power to make her feel comfortable and valued, right? You certainly wouldn't sit in the next room and call out, "Have a seat over there. I'll be with you shortly." And you wouldn't make her sit there for an hour or more with no further acknowledgment of her presence in your home, with no offer of a cool drink nor a clue about where she might find a restroom. If you treated your neighbor that way, can you imagine what she would think (and perhaps even say!) about you after she left? She wouldn't be a raving fan, I can tell you that. You'd gain quite a reputation in the neighborhood, and it wouldn't be a positive one.

I am not saying that a patient coming to your office or clinic is exactly the same as a friend visiting your home. But I am saying that this is a person you have made a commitment to care about. This is a person who is walking into the building you're sitting in because she trusts you with her life. In some cases she is willing to write a giant check to you and the company you work for in exchange for your attention and expert guidance.

Our patients are asking for our help. They're scared. They're confused. They're in pain, and they have no idea how to change that. And what do we do in response? We slide open the little, glass window and order them to go sit down over there, and when we finally decide to let them into our inner sanctum, we treat them like numbers. And then we wonder why they're so frustrated. We wonder why they sue us if even the slightest thing goes wrong. But after we've treated them so poorly, why should we expect them to give us the benefit of the doubt about anything?

There has to be a sea of change in the way we communicate with our patients. But this doesn't mean it has to be difficult or expensive to do so. In this book I am going to give you a ton of quick, simple, cost-effective things you can begin doing *today* to convert Mrs. Smith from a frustrated Code 99242 into a satisfied human being who leaves your office feeling better about her health, about herself, and about her healthcare providers. When that happens Mrs. Smith is going to become a raving patient who uses her voice and today's technology to share the good news about you and your practice with her friends and family.

What follows are proven techniques for great communication, for getting your point across, and for getting people to believe what you say. Many of the methods herein have been used to great positive effect across a variety of industries, and they can be easily applied to a medical practice. Some of the things we'll cover in this book may seem like manipulation, or they may seem like neurolinguistic programming. Admittedly there is some neurolinguistic programming involved in this. But these techniques are not about manipulating patients or influencing them to change according to your whims. They are about communicating in a way that is more likely to have a positive impact. They are about interacting with your patients in a way that helps.

These practical tips and communication techniques are backed up by my personal experience of close to twenty years in medicine and by science and research. I'll cite appropriate studies and provide supporting data just the same as we do in the practice of medicine.

By using the techniques in this book, we will elevate our reputations as individual healthcare providers and as a profession one patient at a time. The goal is that each patient in your care will leave your office feeling satisfied and valued. Each patient will tell another patient about their great experience with you and your staff, and that patient will tell another, and before you know it you will be surrounded by patients who believe in you and who are encouraged by what you have to offer them. The positive news will continue to spread. Eventually your clinic will be packed with people who are on your side — packed with Raving Patients® who want your help, who are willing to follow your instructions to achieve good outcomes, and who are more likely to share their experiences with other quality patients. Patients like these are far less likely to sue you in the event of bad outcomes. When you have happy patients who are making progress and getting better, you will get better too. You'll feel the goodness you're helping to create, and that goodness will carry over into every aspect of your life.

Now is the time to set this in motion. I see the changes that are happening in healthcare today not as frustrating or bad but as opportunities. Change is inevitable, and with these changes will come advances. Because technology continues to evolve so rapidly, we're on the verge of a major breakthrough in the way healthcare will be practiced, and it is electrifying. I am stoked and excited to be a part of it, and you have every reason to be excited too. Our global population is growing and aging, and that means a boom in business. What other industry would be frustrated by that? What other industry wouldn't be licking its chops at the idea of its demographic getting larger and the demand for its services going up? Yet our cynicism and negativity threaten to stand in the way of this growth opportunity. The bottom line is that we can either embrace change and win or fight against it and lose. That's it—there is no other choice. It's like the old saying goes: if you're not part of the solution, you're part of the problem.

The doctor-tested, patient-approved techniques in this book will help you become part of the solution quickly, cost-effectively, and completely. Let's begin.

It Pays to be Nice. Literally.

*Any intelligent fool can make things bigger and
more complex, but it takes a lot of courage
to move in the opposite direction.*

— ALBERT EINSTEIN

Let's say that a sixty-two-year old man named Bob is admitted with chest pain. When we doctors and nurses talk about him amongst ourselves, we don't refer to him as Bob. We call him "the chest pain in room eighty-six." When we get the results of his cardiac panel and get together to decide what the next step will be, his name changes from "the chest pain in room eighty-six" to "the MI in room eighty-six."

You must admit it's true. Too often that is exactly the way we behave. There is no real communication between us and the man named Bob, only a bunch of doctors and nurses standing around looking at numbers and plotting a strategic course as if we were teammates playing a video war game. Video games are easy; anyone — even children — can master them.

But what a child cannot do is understand the nuances of why a particular patient is hurting and what it means to him and his family that he may die. There is a difference in how most of us would communicate with a human being whose life is in danger and "the chest pain in room eighty-six."

Admittedly, a certain amount of detachment is necessary in a case like Bob's. You must maintain control and be a supportive authority figure at a time like that, but there is a fine line between detachment and disconnect. And that is the tightrope we must learn to walk—the balancing act we must work to perfect every single day. How do you learn to serve as both a pillar of support and a comforting shoulder for your patients to lean upon?

The first step is to get over yourself.

The overarching (but basically simple) principal I teach residents and medical students is this:

> *When you are with a patient, you are never the most important person in the room. Ever.*

The best healthcare providers are the ones who live by that maxim of service to their patients. You don't have to get hit by a ton of bricks like I did with a little sick girl and her mom in order to realize this. You can pledge (or renew) your vow of service today. Trust me when I say that everything becomes easier when you stop taking yourself so seriously. Everything becomes more meaningful when you remember you're doing this work to serve others. You are in the customer service business. You are in the sales business. The best customer service people always have the most sales. So step aside and get out of your own way. Step aside and open the door to your patients' trust and cooperation.

You cannot know what is inside a house until you open the door and look around. The same is true with people. You will never really know your patients and be able to serve them well unless you can get them to open the door and let you in. In my experience the key to opening that door is compassionate communication. Once you gain access, you will begin to see the essence of the person you are trying to help, and they will begin to see your essence too. You will begin to see your patients as individuals, and you will become a more effective healthcare provider as a result. Not only that but *research shows that you will be less likely to be sued should something go wrong.*

In a 2002 study conducted by researchers at Harvard, the University of California-Riverside, and the University of Toronto, a team led by Nalini Ambady, PhD, studied 114 audio tapes of 65 surgeons interacting with their patients. Half of the surgeons had been sued for malpractice before; the other half had not. The researchers scored the surgeons on how domineering or kind they were during the first and last minutes of their interactions with the patients. What they discovered was fascinating. The researchers determined that "surgeons' tone of voice in routine visits is associated with malpractice claims history."[2]

In other words surgeons who were rated as domineering and uncaring in their communication with patients were also the surgeons who had been sued the most often for malpractice. Put yet another way, doctors who were more likeable and empathetic in their conversations and dealings with their patients were far less likely to have been sued than their more overbearing peers.

> *The manner or tone in which a physician communicates might be as important to malpractice as what is said. A physician relating to a patient in a "negative" manner (e.g., using a harsh or impatient tone of voice) may trigger litigious feelings when there is a bad result, whereas a physician relating in a "positive" manner may not. Because the medical encounter is often emotionally stressful, patients may be especially sensitive to the emotion communicated by subtle cues such as the tone of voice.*[3]

---

2 Nalini Ambady, Debi LaPlante, Thai Nguyen, Robert Rosenthal, Nigel Chaumeton, Wendy Levinson, "Surgeons' tone of voice: A clue to malpractice history," Surgery 132, 1, accessed December 24, 2012, http://www.wjh.harvard.edu/~na/surgeons%20tone%20of%20voice.pdf.

3 Ambady et al, "Surgeons' tone of voice," 5, 6.

ACTION POINTS

1. *Before entering the room to see the patient, stop and take note of his or her name. Use it in your greeting and in conversation with the patient.*

2. *If you find yourself relating to a patient in a negative manner (i.e. using a harsh or impatient tone of voice), pause and take a proverbial step to the side and begin again in a positive manner. Your malpractice claims history may depend on it.*

3. *Don't take yourself too seriously. Your current frustration will pass. Smile and know everything will work out ten minutes before it's too late.*

4. *Remember that when you are with a patient, you are never the most important person in the room. Ever.*

Universal Characteristics of Friendship

My doctor is nice; every time I see him,
I'm ashamed of what I think of doctors in general.

— MIGNON MCLAUGHLIN

In medicine we're told to establish rapport with the patient. But what exactly does that mean? How do you do that? You do it by becoming the patient's friend for the brief period you are together.

Let me be clear: I am not recommending that you establish a nonmedical relationship. There is a fine line to walk there, and I don't want to be misunderstood. I believe you can maintain a medical relationship and still take certain steps to open yourself up so your patient can see you as an ally and not an enemy. In his excellent book *Unstoppable Confidence: How to Use the Power of NLP to Be More Dynamic and Successful,* author Kent Sayre describes three universal characteristics of friendship that I find particularly applicable to patient care and communication:

- Similarity
- Cooperation
- Praise

Similarity

Friends usually share certain similarities, be they similar physical characteristics or shared interests, activities, values, causes, or worldview. In the typical medical practice, you will probably not be privy to your patients' values and activities, but you can still establish some similarities with them. One way to create a similarity with a patient is through *mirroring*, which means that during your interaction with them, you copy their body language, word usage, gestures, and/or facial expressions. For example you can mirror their position in the chair. If they are leaning forward, then you lean forward. If their legs are crossed, then you cross your legs in the same fashion. If the patient doesn't have anything in their hands, then you set down your chart and empty your hands too. If they raise their eyebrows a lot when they talk, raise your eyebrows when you talk. If they nod, then you nod.

The patient is not likely to pick up on exactly what you are doing, however they will begin to think of you as similar to them. They will see themselves in the mirror of *you*, so to speak, because they're looking at someone who is like them even if it is as subtle as your ankles being crossed in the same way as theirs. This is a *perceived* similarity.

Then there is *true* similarity, which is the more powerful kind. If you find out that a patient collects watches and you do too, bring it up. Ask them about their watch collection. If the patient has a ponytail and you have a ponytail too, then mention it. Say, "Hey, I like your hair!" They'll glance at yours, and now you have something genuine in common. Even if it seems insignificant, you have made a connection. Remember: you cannot have friendship without first making some sort of connection.

Cooperation

The second universal characteristic of a friendship is cooperation, which is critical in a medical practice. People don't visit a doctor because they know everything about their conditions and they feel perfectly fine. Generally there is some sense of confusion within them or they wouldn't be there. They have questions.

At its most basic level, cooperation with patients means seeing to it that those questions are answered quickly, completely, and efficiently. And if you can anticipate what some of their questions might be and answer them up front before they even have to ask, then you will have a head start on the friend-making process.

For example when Mrs. Smith walks into the clinic, she doesn't know where she's going or who will be taking care of her, or what is about to happen. In most clinics the nurse sticks her head into the lobby, calls Mrs. Smith's name, turns around, and starts walking off down the hallway. Mrs. Smith stands up and follows her leader. She doesn't know where she's going. She is simply following someone she doesn't know or relate to at all. That nurse isn't cooperating with her patient; she's expecting her patient to follow blindly. Nobody feels good about being told to follow. If you want to treat people like dogs, then expect them to bark.

But what if Mrs. Smith's visit started like this instead?

"Good morning, Mrs. Smith. I am Rita, Dr. Wonderful's nurse. Welcome to the clinic! Let's walk down this hallway. Oh, I love your dress.... That sunny, yellow color reminds me of springtime. Here on the left is a restroom, just in case. Across the hall is the scale. Let's get your weight, and then we'll head into the examining room on the right, where I'll check your blood pressure and get you settled in for the rest of your visit. Would you like a bottle of water while you wait for Dr. Wonderful?"

Now that's cooperation. That kind of interaction helps the patient. It reduces the unknown. It illuminates the darkness. Be that kind of warm, reassuring light for your patients.

In the case of a follow-up visit, or if there is surgery or a test pending, it is especially important to answer your patients' questions efficiently and clearly. Remember similarity. Your patients probably don't know a lot of medical terms. If you're a nuclear-medicine tech and you're about to do a PET scan and the patient asks you what positron emission technology is, then guess what? You have a question to answer. The best practice is to figure out a good answer *in advance* because if you're in that line of work, you're probably going to be asked that question more than once.

Cooperate with your patients by having an elevator speech ready so you can explain in laymen's terms what it is you're going to do. Answer their questions and fulfill their requests as quickly and efficiently as you can. Find a way to say "yes." That's what friends do.

Praise

There are two ways to see everything: the negative way and the positive way. Friends try to keep things positive when communicating with one another.

"You're morbidly obese," you say to Mr. Smith. "You're getting diabetes. If your diabetes progresses, you're going to have peripheral neuropathy in your toes. You're going to have heart problems. Your vision will deteriorate. You'll continue to be obese, and your blood pressure will continue to climb. You will probably have a heart attack."

Those statements are negative, negative, negative, negative, negative, and negative. Nobody wants to hear that. You're probably thinking, *Well of course they don't want to hear it, but it's true. They're there because they're fat, and they're not headed for a good outcome. They're there because they chose to be that way. I have to tell them the truth!"*

Fair enough. But imagine if I said to the morbidly obese Mr. Smith, "We have an opportunity here, Bob, because you are at a crossroads with your weight. When you get your weight down, you will be able to climb stairs without effort. You will love shopping for new, stylish clothes. You will love the way you look. You will have more energy. You will sleep better. You'll have more strength and vitality, and you'll be able to enjoy Christmases with your grandchildren for many years to come."

Look, your patients already know they're sick and fat. They're not dumb. I'm not saying you must never mention the negatives. I am saying you can convey the truth in such a way that the positives outweigh the negatives. You can mention the high blood pressure and the blood sugar being out of control, but then you can spin it toward the positive.

Stay in the positive whenever you can.

A friend who constantly finds fault with you isn't a friend for long. Nonstop criticism will eventually spell the end of any relationship, be it marriage, friendship, dating, or medicine. Patients are emotionally and mentally breaking up with you in their minds when you're constantly criticizing. Now, I want to qualify this. I am a surgeon, and I understand that if a person chooses to be morbidly obese and smoke and drink heavily, they're going to have horrible problems. There is nothing untrue about what I just said there, but that doesn't change the outcome. You have an opportunity to reframe things for your patients by shifting conversations into a positive context and nudging them forward. Stopping them in their tracks with criticism isn't going to help them. It's only going to make your patients feel bad and earn you a reputation as a world-class jerk.

So the next time you're discussing smoking with a patient and he says, "I know, I know. You're going to tell me I need to quit smoking…again," you can reply, "No, I'm not. Not today. You can continue smoking if you wish. This is America. You have that right. I'm only telling you what you can achieve without smoking and how your life will be better moving forward. You *can* quit — it is not as hard as the tobacco industry would like you to believe. Bob, I know you. With your guts and determination, I know you can do it. And when you quit smoking, you will be able to throw the football around with your kids, and maybe even play a little pickup basketball too."

People respect that. Now they have a choice. Now they've received praise. You've cooperated with them. So if a patient has lost five pounds, don't say, "Well, you need to lose seventy more." Say, "Fantastic! That is five pounds fewer than you weighed last time. And do you realize that your blood pressure is lower this time too? Now *that's* progress! Keep going!"

Everybody loves praise. Keep your interactions with patients positive, and watch your fan base expand exponentially.

ACTION POINTS

1. *Establish similarity through mirroring. Mirror body language, word usage, gestures, and facial expressions to establish perceived similarity.*

2. *If you and your patient have a true similarity, mention it. Use it as a starting point for building trust and patient confidence.*

3. *Anticipate common questions and prepare answers that will put your patients at ease. Cooperate in your patients' care by reducing the unknown for them.*

4. *Choose to provide positive suggestions rather than negative criticism. Illustrate the positive outcomes and benefits of your recommendations.*

Dunbar's Number

*In the sick room, ten cents' worth of human understanding
equals ten dollars' worth of medical science.*

— MARTIN H. FISCHER

With rare exceptions each human being has an innate need to
associate and engage in fellowship with others. Back in ancient
times, we formed clans to satisfy that need. Today our family
members, close friends, neighbors, colleagues, and others with
whom we are close make up our modern-day clans. But there is a
limit to the number of people with whom we can maintain stable
social relations. As it turns out, that limit is not arbitrary. It is set
by our brains.

According to Robin Dunbar, professor of evolutionary anthro-
pology at the University of Oxford, the human brain is hardwired
in a way that restricts the number of friendships we can maintain
at any given time. That average number—known as Dunbar's
number—is approximately 150. Therefore we humans can handle only reciprocal, meaningful relationships with around 150
people. Dunbar's research shows this was true back in the cave-
man days and it is also true today.

Consider the Facebook phenomenon. People friend you, you
friend them back, and then you don't talk to them for years. So

while you may have a thousand Facebook "friends," you probably really communicate with less than one hundred of them on a monthly basis. Or think of how many Christmas cards you send on average. Probably around one hundred. Your Christmas card list is your Dunbar's number. These are the people in your life whom you trust. People you appreciate. People you praise and receive praise from, and people you would help in a crisis. I'm not talking about pulling somebody you don't know out of a burning building. We should all do that. I'm talking about if my friend Joe has a problem, then I'm there for him. I want to help him. It's my moral obligation to do so because Joe is one of my Dunbar's numbers. He is part of my clan. I may read about something bad happening to a person I don't know who lives on the other side of the state, and while I feel empathy for her I'm probably not going to drive to her house and bring her a pan of lasagna. She's not one of my Dunbar's numbers. She is not in my clan. But if my pal Joe broke his leg, I would drive over and deliver a pan of lasagna and probably even rake his yard while I was there.

Now, why is this important for you to know as a healthcare provider? Because if you can become one of Dunbar's numbers for your patients, they will be more likely to listen to what you say. They will be more likely to follow your recommendations. They will be more likely to appreciate you and to tell other people in their clan about you. They'll be less likely to sue you. Therefore your goal is to create a relationship with each patient so they see you as one of their Dunbar's numbers. Obviously this is more likely to happen in primary-care situations in which patients visit a particular healthcare provider on a regular basis.

Make an effort to communicate with all patients in such a way that they can absorb what you're saying. Strive to communicate in such a way that they view you as someone who is similar to them in some way. Ask about their families and friends. Ask about hobbies, pastimes, last weekend, or their favorite sports teams. Parents are proud of their children. Ask and they will tell you so. Strangers don't ask you about your kids. People in your Dunbar's number do. People in your Dunbar's number care about you and your interests.

Whenever you show your patients that you care, in their minds you are dialing in to their clan. You are dialing in to their Dunbar's number. They will think of you when they need something or when they want to provide value to another person. If a friend needs a referral to a good doctor, guess what? They will say, "You know, Dr. Wonderful is excellent. You can't go wrong with her. That's who I go to, and I think she's just great."

> *When things do not go as expected, patients are less likely to be aggressive, judgmental, and litigious to those in their Dunbar's number.*

Again, I am not suggesting that you have to establish nonmedical relationships with your patients in order to become one of their Dunbar's numbers. Simply be on the lookout for opportunities to be more trustworthy, more approachable, more reliable, more positive, more empathetic, and more compassionate whenever you're in the company of your patients. You and your growing clan of Raving Patients® will be very happy that you did.

ACTION POINTS

1. *Be on the lookout for opportunities to be more positive, empathetic, interested, compassionate, and approachable. Make an effort to join your patient's Dunbar's number.*

2. *Mention and capitalize on a nonmedical similarity you have with the patient.*

3. *If your friend breaks his leg, bring him a pan of lasagna.*

Choose Your Perception

Treat the patient, not the X-ray.

—James M. Hunter

In his book *Blink*, author Malcolm Gladwell writes that we tend to make judgments of others within the first ten seconds of meeting them. When we do that, we are forming perceptions based upon...well, not much of anything concrete and meaningful. Those snap perceptions—which are sometimes dead wrong—have a powerful influence on the way we communicate with one another. If you want to communicate effectively with your patients (and I know you do!) then you must recognize this tendency in yourself and gain control of it.

The good news is that you can stop making faulty, impulsive judgments about other people and learn to communicate from a place of openness and truth. You do that by setting an intention to be positive until there is an established need to be otherwise—to be receptive to whoever the other person truly is and not to how they might appear at first glance. Before you open the examining-room door, you have the opportunity—no, the responsibility—to create a firm intention to connect with the patient and project an image of sincerity, openness, and compassion. By doing so you essentially turn on the light in the room when you walk inside. You increase the likelihood that you will end up helping that patient.

But not if you do as so many of us in medicine unfortunately do. Not if you say to yourself, "Next I have to see the fat guy in room three." It's cruel and horrible to say, but that's the way far too many of us think and behave. When you do that, you've already perceived that person negatively. You've already allowed a seed to sprout in your mind that something is wrong with that person, and you're starting a medical relationship based upon that negativity. You don't know anything about the man, but in your mind he's the fat guy in room three. You have chosen a negative perception.

Unfortunately I have firsthand experience with this. I am not proud to share this story (especially as the author of a book like this one), but for the sake of making my point, it's self-disclosure time:

One night several years ago, I was called to the emergency room at about three o'clock on a Monday morning to treat a male patient who had been involved in a violent assault in a bar with a broken beer bottle. The man had been in the United States for only about two months. He spoke very little English and had no insurance. My immediate perception was that he must have been doing something wrong. After all he had been involved in an assault late at night. He was from out of the country. And since he didn't have insurance, I knew I was never going to get paid. In my mind this was what we call in the surgery business a classic "dump." I was convinced of it before I even got in my car. When I arrived at the emergency room, I was all attitude with a perception of disdain for being called at 3:00 a.m. Disdain is not a characteristic that endears you to the nursing staff upon whom you will rely for help. Just FYI.

I spent two hours in the emergency room repairing the cuts on this man's face—cuts that ran across his jawbone and down into his lips. He was accompanied by a cousin who spoke a little bit of English, so I wrote instructions for them to come see me in a week so we could remove the sutures. I was certain I would never see this patient again. I was frustrated because I had just done two hours of surgery for free.

Well, imagine my surprise when a week later—exactly at the time I had asked them to come back—the man and his cousin showed up. They walked into my office wearing very nice suits; in fact they looked far nicer than I did that day. In broken English the patient apologized to the receptionist for his inability to communicate well and told her that his cousin would be speaking for him and filling out his forms for the duration of his visit.

So they went down the hallway into the examination room, and my assistant took out the sutures. When I went in, the cousin thanked me profusely for helping them through such a traumatic event the week before. Then he asked for the amount of my bill. My assistant went out to the front desk and found out what the charges would be if we were submitting a bill to insurance. We wrote that amount down on a slip of paper and handed it to the patient, who promptly reached into his coat pocket, pulled out a roll of hundred-dollar bills, and paid me on the spot. In full.

My perception about that man had been totally wrong. I was completely aghast and embarrassed once I realized my mistake. He was not a bad person after all—he was a decent human being who wanted to do right by me. I never shared my prejudgments (and my resulting feelings of shame) with that patient. I don't know if I should have or not.

That is the damage that stereotypes and prejudices do in our society. They alter our perceptions. They muddy the waters and adversely influence the way we treat other people. But when we learn to move forward without judgment regarding religion, nationality, creed, skin color, weight, sexuality, language, etc., everything becomes clearer. When you train yourself to automatically perceive the patient as a kind person who needs your help rather than "the fat guy in room three" or "the deadbeat criminal in the ER," then you will project positivity and warmth when you walk in. When you learn to instinctively think of the patient as someone who is frightened and is in physical and/or emotional pain, you will be more likely to help that person. You'll be more likely to give thoughtful answers to their questions. You'll be more likely to fulfill your responsibility to provide them with the best care possible.

When you begin the conversation in a positive tone, the patient will be more likely to respond in a positive fashion. But if you walk into the exam room with your brow furrowed, thinking, *This guy is an ass; he was rude to the front-desk people because he had to wait for an hour, and now he's going to take it out on me too*, then the chances are pretty good that your perception will be correct. That patient probably *is* going to be a jerk to you largely because you are projecting a negative attitude of your own and he perceives it. Nobody is going to have a good outcome now.

Allow me to return for a moment to the point of the proverbial deadbeat criminal in the ER. I am not too clueless to know that sometimes a negative preconception is, in fact, correct. Sometimes the patient *is* an ass and you won't get paid. Do the right thing anyway, and do it for two reasons. Number one: you will know you did the right thing. You can go home and sleep at night knowing you treated someone with respect despite it being very difficult to do so. Number two: someone else will always be watching you. Your coworkers, your assistants, and other bystanders will be impressed by how you handled such a difficult situation. When you handle a situation with class, dignity, and calm confidence, those observing you will be effusive in their praise of you to others. Do it for the referrals, for your reputation, and for the public-relations boost it can be for your career.

At the beginning of every single interaction, you have the power to choose your perception and set your intention before you walk in the room. You can either set an intention of defending yourself or you can intend to defuse a potentially difficult situation. Don't intend to defend. Our patients aren't there to storm the castle. They're there to help build it. So sitting up in your guard tower expecting someone you haven't even met yet to shoot arrows at you is a total waste of energy. Don't go in with that kind of attitude. Pick a positive intention instead, and walk in projecting that. Make the first ten seconds with your patients memorable for all the right reasons.

ACTION POINTS

1. *Before every patient interaction, choose a positive perception of what you expect to happen with that patient.*

2. *When you are called in at an inconvenient time, leave your negative attitude behind. You just might get paid in full — in cash.*

3. *Even if you are in a less than ideal interaction, remember someone is watching you. Stay positive and act professionally. Your reputation depends on it.*

Comfort and Ease

A physician is obligated to consider more than a diseased organ, more even than the whole man — he must view the man in his world.

— HARVEY CUSHING

In order to communicate with you, your patients need to be comfortable in your presence. This is admittedly a vague term. But I can tell you from personal experience that sitting up on a high table in a cold room, naked except for a crinkly paper gown, is not comfortable. It doesn't put you at ease. Neither does sitting in a low chair while a six-foot-five doctor towers over you with a scowl punching out notes on the computer tablet in his hand.

When you first approach each and every patient, think about what would provide the most physical comfort for that person. When you stand or sit behind a patient in a wheelchair so she has to turn her head and crank her shoulders around in order to see you or to answer your questions, then your patient is not comfortable in your presence. Move around to the front of the wheelchair and sit or kneel down at that patient's level to talk to her. It doesn't take any more time to do that.

And on the occasions when you can't make things more comfortable, at least acknowledge the patient's discomfort.

"Well, obviously this exam gown isn't going to win any fashion awards, but we need you to put it on anyway. I know it's uncomfortable. If you could just sit up here on the table for a moment, we're going to get this examination out of the way. We'll be as quick and gentle as we can, I promise."

There—you've just made that patient more comfortable. She's still doing an unpleasant thing. She's still sitting up on a high table, naked except for a paper gown, but at least you've made an effort to ease her mind a little bit.

Remember that it's uncomfortable for a patient to have to turn their head to one side or the other to talk to you, so sit in front of them at their level. Looking straight down or straight up is hard for many people, so if you're showing them a chart, illustration, or lab result, move it in front of them and hold it so they can see it easily. The most comfortable area is about nine inches up or down from the level of their eyes.

These are some simple ways to make patients more at ease physically. When that occurs there is emotional comfort. Offer a kind word. Shake their hand. Provide some praise. Find or establish some similarity between the two of you. Answer their questions. Smile. If you don't feel like smiling, that's your problem. That's not the patient's problem. So smile even if you have to fake it because that's what it's going to take to make the patient feel more comfortable in your presence. And if you fake it long enough, the chances are very good that your patient will give you a legitimate reason to smile before your visit is over. Trust me on that.

Making someone comfortable in your presence doesn't have to be a long, convoluted, drawn-out process. It's the small, thoughtful, common-sense things that make the biggest impact. Practice makes perfect.

ACTION POINTS

1. *Position yourself in front of the patient at their eye level. Help them achieve a comfortable body position in order to listen better to your recommendations.*

2. *Acknowledge an uncomfortable situation for the patient with reassurance and gratitude for their cooperation.*

3. *Smile more.*

The Eyes Have It

To me the ideal doctor would be a man endowed with profound knowledge of life and of the soul, intuitively divining any suffering or disorder of whatever kind, and restoring peace by his mere presence.

—HENRI AMIEL

As a surgeon and a medical educator for many years now, I can tell you from experience that making eye contact with patients is critical to establishing a healthy medical relationship. In fact nonverbal communication (including eye contact) in a clinical setting has been called "the channel most responsible for communicating attitudes, emotions, and affect."[4]

It's just common sense, isn't it? When someone looks you in the eye, you can see that they are communicating their interest in you. They are showing you that they respect you as a person. When someone doesn't look you in the eye, they are indicating that you don't matter very much. That they may not be trustworthy. That they are not listening intently. Making eye contact is a

4 M.R. DiMatteo, A. Taranta, H.S. Friedman, L.M. Prince, "Predicting patient satisfaction from physicians' nonverbal communication skill," *Med Care* 18, 4 (1980):376–387, accessed January 1, 2013, www.ncbi.nlm.nih.gov/pmc/articles/PMC2814257/.

way to put people at ease and establish rapport and trust. We all know this, yet it is amazing to me how many doctors don't make an effort to establish eye contact with their patients. I'm not talking about staring into someone's eyes and never blinking. That's called Parkinson's disease. I'm simply talking about looking someone in the eye when you're asking them questions or making a medical recommendation or giving them a diagnosis. It's vitally important to your success, and I'm not the only one who thinks so. Study after study proves it.

Take, for instance, a 2009 study[5] by Taiwanese researchers in which they measured the amount of time that doctors maintained eye contact with patients during medical consultations. The study showed that the patients who received more eye contact from their doctors "scored a higher level of verbal participation" than those who received less. In other words the study concluded that eye contact by the doctors "encourages patients' narration of their health problems."

Simply put, patients share more information when their doctors look them in the eye more often.

Establishing frequent eye contact is vitally important in every aspect of our lives, yet we're getting worse and worse at it. Technology is one of the major culprits. Rather than looking at the people around us, we stare at our tablets, our laptops, and our phones. Think about the average teenager. You're trying to talk to your child, but he is looking at his phone and mumbling, "Yeah, Mom, OK, OK." And how do you respond? You instantly order him to stop what he's doing and look at you because you haven't established eye contact. You don't feel confident that he is listening to you. He *may* be listening, but unless his eyeballs are pointed in your direction, you are not sure he is getting your message. That is Basic Human Interaction 101, and it is just as important in the examining room as it is around the kitchen table.

---

5 Shu-fen Cheng, Feng-hwa Lu, "Eye Contact as a Nonverbal Strategy in Facilitating Patients' Verbal Participation," accessed January 1, 2013, http:// faculty.ksu.edu.sa/aljarf/Documents/MDALL%20conference%202009%20 -%20language%20and%20linguistics/02.pdf.

If you are with a patient but you're focused on charting something on your tablet, then you are no different from the kid with the smartphone in his hand whose mom wants his undivided attention. "Put down the phone and look at me!" she shouts in exasperation. Well, guess what? That's what your patient wants to say to you. *Put down the tablet and look at me, Doctor. For heaven's sake, at least make eye contact!*

If you have an important point to make, make it with your eyes first. Put down the device and speak with your eyes and your hands. Don't point, but do make gestures. Hand motions and eye contact are like exclamation points in writing. Use them to drive home your message and to show your patients that you are completely engaged and one hundred percent present. They deserve nothing less from you.

ACTION POINTS

1. *Structure your consultations to include sufficient time for charting and for active patient engagement, including eye contact.*

2. *During the most vital portions of your discussion about diagnosis, findings, and treatment, make certain to establish eye contact with the patient.*

3. *Determine the patient's eye color. When you know the color of your patient's eyes, you will know that you have established adequate eye contact.*

The Pratfall Effect

Laughter is the tonic, the relief, the surcease for pain.

— CHARLIE CHAPLIN

It's like your mom always said — nobody's perfect. We all make mistakes. Nobody is immune. Still, those of us working in the healthcare profession generally work hard to avoid making errors because patients' lives are on the line and because we want to protect our reputations. Many of us do that by creating an air of superiority about ourselves. We walk into the examining room with the appearance of one who knows everything, one who is going to tell the patient how it's going to be. We know in our hearts that we're not perfect, but we're going to do whatever we can to make everyone *think* we are. No human frailties allowed.

But did you know that exhibiting a foible every now and then can actually be good for patient relations? It's true according to a research paper published in 1966 by Elliot Aronson, et al. The abstract for the paper, entitled "The Effect of a Pratfall on Increasing Interpersonal Attractiveness," states as follows:

> *An experiment was performed which demonstrated that the attractiveness of a superior person is enhanced if he commits a clumsy blunder; the same blunder tends to decrease the attractiveness of a*

mediocre person. These results were predicted by conjecturing that a superior person may be viewed as superhuman and, therefore, distant; a blunder tends to humanize him and, consequently, increases his attractiveness.[6]

Aronson called this phenomenon "the pratfall effect" and summed it up by writing that when a competent person makes a mistake and shows vulnerability, he becomes more likable to others. The physical pratfall has been used in comedy for centuries because let's face it—it's funny. People laugh at pratfalls every time because we can all relate to them. Every single one of us has stumbled at one time or another.

In his book *59 Seconds: Think a Little, Change a Lot,* author Richard Wiseman tells how he tested the pratfall effect. He set up an experiment in a shopping mall and rounded up a group of shoppers to participate. An assembled crowd was told by Wiseman and his crew that those in the crowd would be watching demonstrations by two young women trainees on how to make a fruit juice concoction in a new blender. The first to perform her demonstration was Sara, who played the role of the superior person. Sara had already spent much time practicing with the blender and had perfected a compelling verbal presentation for her demo. She performed flawlessly, and the audience gave her a rousing round of applause.

Next was Emma, who was to play the role of the bumbler. When she put the fruit in the blender and turned it on, the lid blew off and Emma was doused by fruit. Feigning embarrassment, she poured what remained of the blender's contents into a glass and received the crowd's empathetic applause.

Wiseman and his colleagues then asked the audience which demonstration and which demonstrator appealed to them the most. The participants said that while they thought Sara's

---

6 Elliot Aronson, Ben Willerman, Joanne Floyd, "The effect of a pratfall on increasing interpersonal attractiveness," *Psychonomic Science* 4, 6 (1966), 227–228, accessed January 7, 2012, http://psycnet.apa.org/psycinfo/1966-05356-001.

demonstration was the most proficient and compelling, they liked Emma more because they could relate to her better.

Whenever I think of the pratfall effect, I immediately think of the late, great chef Julia Child. One of the chief reasons Julia's cooking shows were so popular was that she appeared to be so normal, meaning she made a lot of mistakes. She did not seem like the stereotypical aloof French chef. Julia was a fine cook, but she was always dropping things, cutting herself, flipping the omelet all wrong, making enormous messes in the studio kitchen.... In other words she let herself be real in front of us, and we loved her for it. We could relate to her. Julia's willingness to be seen as clumsy turned her into a cultural icon.

If you're a doctor or nurse, a small slipup during your verbal interaction makes you more approachable. It tears down the emotional barrier that naturally exists between the superior person (you, the healthcare provider) and the patient. The doctor appears more accessible to the patient after making a small blunder. I'm not saying that you should enter the room and do a Chevy Chase-style pratfall — that would make you look like a goof — but the occasional small slipup can enhance your likability and bring you closer to your patient.

For example a few years ago I recommended surgery for a particular patient. As I described the procedure to her, I accidently dropped the pen I had been using. As I stooped to pick it up, I said, "Wow! I'll bet *that* boosts your confidence in your surgeon, eh?" The patient instantly cracked up. My blooper diffused the tension. It made me seem much less intimidating. You may not be surprised to know that as a consequence, I fumble my pen more often than I used to. Just sayin'.

On another occasion I noticed during a consultation that I had a small blotch of peanut butter on my shirt sleeve. Instead of trying to hide it, I drew attention to it.

"Oops!" I chuckled as I wiped the spot away. "Looks like my daughter's peanut butter toast got the best of me when I was making her breakfast this morning!" My patient chuckled along with me and nodded knowingly.

That kind of pratfall enhances your reputation; it does not detract from it.

In our education and training as healthcare professionals, we're taught to know every answer. Our only expectation is perfection, and that becomes our goal. But when you break that mold a little bit, it makes you more human to your patients. They'll be more likely to buy what you're selling, which is health and wellness, and they'll be less likely to see you as an adversary should something go seriously wrong.

ACTION POINTS

1. *Don't be afraid to let patients see that you are not perfect. It makes you seem more human and less intimidating.*

2. *With discretion, acknowledge a small foible as it happens. Research shows this will likely put the patient at ease and help him or her to see you as likeable.*

Set a Great Example

Never forget that it is not a pneumonia,
but a pneumonic man who is your patient.

—William Withey Gull

Would you trust an obese personal trainer to help you get in shape? Would you have confidence in a smoking cessation expert who comes back from her breaks smelling like an ashtray? How about a nutritionist who gorges on greasy fast food every day for lunch, or a marriage counselor who has been divorced three times? Of course you wouldn't trust them. You can't take a person seriously when they don't bother to practice what they preach.

We all know that the single best thing we can do as a parent, as an employer, as a spouse, as a friend, or as a healthcare provider is to set a great example. You can never question the motives of those who make themselves examples of what they recommend. The video has to match the audio, so to speak. There is no faking that—at least not for long.

Unfortunately many healthcare professionals are out of sync when it comes to setting proper examples. I've been in maternity wards with my own kids where the neonatal nurses smelled like smoke. I can't imagine that is the example they would like to set for their tiny patients and their young parents. I can name two cardiologists right now who are morbidly obese. For the life of me, I can't understand how they expect their patients to follow their recommendations when they don't even follow them themselves. That would be like telling my children they should treat other people with respect but then immediately turning around and being rude to the waiter. Suddenly I am not a credible role model anymore.

This is also true in your relationships with the people who work in your office. If you're a physician and you are disrespectful to the front desk person, the PA, or the nurse, then guess what? They're going to be disrespectful to the patients and they're probably going to be snippy with you too. It all comes down to setting an example. If you go the extra mile with your patients and the people in your office see that, they will go the extra mile with your patients as well, and everyone will be happier. It is like a snowball rolling downhill. The goodness will just grow and grow.

Please don't think this is just a bunch of warm and fuzzy Kumbaya drum-circle silliness. Research shows that creating a work environment characterized by mutual respect *will actually make your business more profitable*! In a *Harvard Business Review* study from 2000[7], researcher Daniel Goleman found that the way employees feel about how their managers and bosses treat them (the corporate climate) *accounts for at least one-third of a company's profitability*. That's no joke.

As the leader you have to be the one to start that happy (and lucrative) snowball rolling. You have to set the tone by setting a good example. You have to take the initiative and go to work every day with the expectation that you're going to make a positive difference for your people and your patients. When you go in with that expectation, then that is what you exude. When you approach each colleague, employee, and patient with the idea that you're going to set a proper example for each of them, then that

---

7 Daniel Goleman, "Leadership That Gets Results," *Harvard Business Review*, March-April 2000.

is what you will do. If you're going to tell someone to be nice to the patients, then for heaven's sake, you be nice too.

If you're going to tell someone to exercise, then tell them how much *you* exercise. If you're going to make a recommendation about their diet, then tell them about your favorite healthy meal. There is nothing wrong with that. That kind of self-disclosure crosses no professional line of demarcation. That is what's called *connecting with the patient*, and it is your business to do that.

Set a proper example in your appearance, in the way you speak, and in the way you treat other people. That's important for any healthcare professional to do. For example there's a stereotype of pediatricians—that they wear silly cartoon-character ties and buttons and things like that because it puts their little patients at ease. A three-year-old who sees SpongeBob on her doctor's tie is probably going to smile. She's probably going to feel better. She's probably going to open up and be okay with what her doctor does and says.

Now, the flip side of that is the neurosurgeon who walks into a consultation wearing a poorly knotted SpongeBob tie and mismatched socks under his scruffy Birkenstocks. That's an example you don't want to set. If you can't tie a tie, how can you tie a suture around my aneurysm? You must always think about the example you're setting for your patients. Look like a professional.

I once heard a lecture given by Thomas Rhodes, general counsel for the American Academy of Facial Plastic and Reconstructive Surgery, and I wrote down something he said because it really resonated with me. He said, "You're always better off wearing a white coat than wearing gold chains."

There is a lot of truth to that. You must always look the part. You have to set an example for what it means to be a healthcare professional. Gold chains, tight T-shirts, sandals, careless grooming.... In my opinion these have no place in a medical practice—at least not if you want your patients to respect you. Right now you may be thinking that people shouldn't judge others on their appearances. After all we cannot judge our patients that way, so why should they be able to judge us? That's fine. You can think that if you wish, but it isn't the reality. Our patients *do* judge us on our appearances. They *do* judge the words we say. They *do* judge us on whether we make eye contact or not and on the way we treat others. That's the honest truth.

So strive to set a great example in all aspects of your behavior, demeanor, and appearance. Hold your staff to those same high standards as well. You can't go wrong if you do.

ACTION POINTS

1. *Set an example for your patients by demonstrating with your actions what you recommend for them.*

2. *Communicate your example to your patients. For example discuss your favorite healthy meals, your exercise routine, or how you quit a bad habit. Your recommendations will be much more believable, and your patients will be far more likely to follow them.*

3. *Interact with your patients in the way you would like your co-workers or employees to interact with your patients.*

4. *Set an example with your appearance. Dress professionally.*

The Accidental Compliment

Each patient ought to feel somewhat the better
after the physician's visit, irrespective of the nature
of the illness.

—WARFIELD THEOBALD LONGCOPE

Flattering another person is a tricky undertaking. When someone issues an over-the-top compliment that surpasses the boundaries of reality, it makes the giver look bad and the receiver feel even worse. It makes you question the giver's motives. But heartfelt praise delivered with skill and sincerity is a terrific way to bring two people together. Therefore it is a talent every healthcare provider should master according to a 2010 article in *The Lancet* by Anthony L. Black, et al.:

> *Physicians tend to overlook praise as part of the communication repertoire. Although we acknowledge that praise has received little attention empirically, we think praise deserves special mention because we find that, if used judiciously, praise is a powerful tool that*

can help deepen conversation and enable physician and patient to move through difficult conversations.[8]

In her excellent book *How to Talk to Anyone: 92 Little Tricks for Big Success in Relationships,* author Leil Lowndes offers tips for giving praise and compliments that unite the giver and the receiver. One way is to make it look as if an admiring comment just slipped out by accident. For example if you are speaking with a patient and in the midst of a sentence you interrupt yourself to say, "Hey, that's a really pretty bracelet, by the way," that comes across as a heartfelt, genuine thought. It does not appear to be forced or contrived. So when you are speaking with a patient and you notice something positive about them, stop in mid-sentence and tell them. Mention how nice their hair looks. Compliment their weight loss. Speak up if you notice they are wearing a cool necklace or if you like their boots. Don't be afraid. Giving a compliment is like putting a coin in the Good Feelings Meter. You're adding a few extra moments of positive regard to that relationship every time you do it.

"Hello Mrs. Smith! Thank you so much for coming in today. Let's head down this hallway to the first door on the left. Gosh, I love that handbag—it is fabulous! OK, here we are...."

That kind of spontaneity shows that you're human—that you're not just there to spout off a bunch of technical information and tap on your iPad and walk out the door. You are there to look at and talk with the patient. You are there to engage with them. Show it by sneaking a little sincere praise into your sentences every now and then.

Another great technique is to talk about your patient behind his back. Now obviously I am not advocating that you participate in hurtful gossip. I'm advocating that you say something nice about your patient to someone else, but make sure the patient

---

8 Anthony L. Back, Robert M. Arnold, Walter F. Baile, Kelly A. Edwards, James A. Tulsky, "When praise is worth considering in a difficult conversation," *The Lancet* 376, 9744 (September 11, 2010): 866–867, accessed January 8, 2013, www.thelancet.com/journals/lancet/article/PIIS0140-6736(10)61401-8/.

can overhear you. For instance as you're walking out of the examining room after seeing a patient, you can say to a nurse in the hallway, "Wow, Mrs. Smith is such a fun lady! You are going to love her!" or "You know what? Terrific patients like Bob Smith make me love coming to work every day. He's a stand-up guy."

Give those kinds of behind-the-back compliments often, and don't be shy about it. Let those patients hear them. Let everybody hear them. It's a great way to forge a deeper, more positive connection with your patients. Try it with your coworkers too. It's a nice way to boost everyone's confidence and foster greater teamwork.

ACTION POINTS

1. *When you notice something positive about the patient (weight loss, hairstyle, handbag, etc.), mention it even if you are mid-sentence. A spontaneous compliment is taken as heartfelt and genuine and helps you engage with the patient.*

2. *If you say something complimentary about your patient to someone else, allow the patient you are complimenting to overhear you.*

3. *When your employee or colleague does something positive, compliment them and let other people hear it. Compliments boost confidence and foster teamwork.*

Write It Down

Some patients, though conscious that their condition is perilous, recover their health simply through their contentment with the goodness of the physician.

— HIPPOCRATES

You've probably been in an interview or some other business encounter in which you said something to the interviewer and she suddenly stopped and wrote down whatever it was you said. Instantly you thought, *Wow…that must have been an important point!* When somebody breaks eye contact with you to write something down, or when they nod while you're talking and then stop to jot a note, they have acknowledged that your words mattered to them. And that's a good feeling.

That's why I recommend that you do the same thing for your patients. If a patient says something positive such as, "I lost ten pounds since the last time I was here," then stop, raise your eyebrows, nod, and write it down. Write it on a piece of scratch paper. Write it on the back cover of whatever you're holding. I don't care if you write it on the gum wrapper in your pocket. What you write it on doesn't matter. What matters is that they see the physical motion of you recording their words. The fact that you've acknowledged what they said as a positive and that you made a point of writing it down—that's their prize. Simply nodding your head in agreement is not nearly as powerful an action as stopping to write it down.

It is important to note that this pertains only to positive statements. Don't let them see you recording negative things. People feel threatened when they say something like, "I'm smoking more than I ever have" and then they see you stop to write that down. That's like being in the principal's office. You're intimidating them. You're accentuating a negative. Accentuate the positive instead by taking down a quick note in front of your patient. They will see that you think their words are important, and they'll appreciate your acknowledgment.

ACTION POINTS

1. *Track your conversations for positives and write notes about them in front of the patient.*

2. *Minimize your reaction to disappointing negatives. Writing down a negative comment will make the patient feel as if they are in trouble.*

Would Someone Please Get the Phone?

Politeness and consideration for others
is like investing pennies and getting dollars back.

— THOMAS SOWELL

I should probably write an entire book about best practices for healthcare professionals who speak with patients over the telephone. It's that important. Why? Because in most cases, a telephone call is the first contact a patient has with your office. It is your first opportunity to make a good impression. Don't blow it! The way that call is conducted will set the tone for the entire patient experience going forward. You want that tone to be positive and pleasant. Here's how to make it so:

In the broadcasting industry, there is an old axiom that says that to sound normal over the radio, you have to project more enthusiasm than is comfortable. I've done radio voiceovers myself, and I can vouch for that. I felt like a complete fool because of the exaggerated, theatrical way I had to speak in order to sound good on the radio. But when the tape was played back for me later, I was shocked to find that my voice was totally appropriate and sounded positive.

The telephone is the same way. You have to find ways to make up for the fact that the person on the other end of the line cannot

assess your body language cues—your appearance, your demeanor, your nodding head, your hand gestures. There is no eye
contact. You have nothing to help you in the conversation except
your voice. Therefore you must accentuate your voice beyond
normal when you talk to someone on the phone.

If someone calls to make an appointment, throw in as many
positive words and exclamations as you can. Check out the difference between these two examples:

"Good morning. Yes, we have an appointment for you. We'll
see you at three."

Or…

"Good morning, Janet! Thank you for calling. Yes, we certainly do have an appointment for you. Three o'clock, yes, absolutely! See you then!"

The first example communicates boredom. The second example conveys enthusiasm and friendliness. I recognize that it
feels weird to inject that many exclamations into your speech. I
understand that it may be difficult for many people to do. One
great trick for keeping your enthusiasm level high is to keep a
mirror on your desk and look at your reflection when you're talking on the phone. If you look bored, you sound bored. If you
look mad, you sound mad. Practice appearing to be happy. Smile.
When you smile while you're talking, that smile is conveyed in
the words you say and in the inflection of your voice.

Talk with your hands even though the patient can't see you.
Talking with your hands will boost your enthusiasm level and
actively communicate your pleasure at speaking with that patient. Use your voice and your words to let them know you are
glad they called. There is absolutely nothing wrong with using a
brief scripted telephone greeting, especially for ancillary phone
staff who may not be accustomed to working with patients on
the phone very often. There are some specialties where it's not so
comfortable for patients to talk about what's wrong with them
over the phone. Who wants to call in and be forced to share the
intimate details of their yeast infection with an unskilled receptionist? In particular, if yours is a plastic surgery office, a urology
office, or a gynecology clinic, do your patients a favor and write

down some scripted examples of phrases that are designed to diffuse discomfort, and keep them by the phone. Show your patients that you're there to help, not to judge.

Before letting a caller go, always thank them for calling. They have made an effort to connect with you. They are taking time out of their busy day for that call, and their time is just as valuable as yours. Acknowledge that truth by being positive and over-the-top. You will get a better response and much more respect from callers when you do.

And finally a word about answering machines…. OK, three words: *I hate them.* Someone calls a doctor's office for personal care, and the first thing they hear is a cold, robotic machine? For heaven's sake, nobody wants to talk to a machine! Having an answering machine sends the signal that you don't value your patients enough to hire a human being to take care of them on the telephone. "Your call is important to us…just not important enough for us to actually talk to you. Please remain on the line, and when we feel like communicating with a patient and allowing you to pay our mortgages for us, your call will be answered in the order in which it was received."

Obviously I just opened a can of sarcasm on you, but you get my point. If your practice is so busy that you think you need to have an answering machine, then wallow in gratitude for being that busy, and forget about the machine. There is probably a very good reason why you're so busy, and it's probably that you have the right person—a human—answering your phone.

ACTION POINTS

1. *Mystery shop at your front desk. Have an anonymous friend call in to ask a few questions, then get their feedback on how it went. Use that feedback to devise ways to improve the telephone experience for your patients.*

2. *Have an in-service training on telephone etiquette so everyone on staff understands how to handle phone calls.*

3. *Forego any automated answering machine and have a kind, helpful human answer your phone.*

4. *Over-animate and accentuate your conversational style when you are on the phone. You and your staff will sound far more positive and eager to help your patients.*

Acknowledge Frustration

Better than a thousand hollow words,
is one word that brings peace.

— BUDDHA

If you ever want to watch frustration go from simmer to steam to a full rolling boil, hang out in a medical office waiting room for an afternoon. Sure, there's a nice little sign on the wall that says, "If it is fifteen minutes after your scheduled appointment, please let someone know!" but the reality is that the sign usually doesn't mean a thing. I know from personal experience, because I've been a patient in a waiting room with such a sign. It was way past my appointment, so I got up and tapped on the receptionist's sliding window.

"Excuse me, hello!" I said with a smile. "Your sign says to let you know if it's fifteen minutes after my scheduled appointment. So here I am, letting you know. Actually it's twenty minutes past my appointment time."

"Yes," she replied. "We'll be with you in a minute or two."

And I thought, *No, you won't.*

To put it bluntly, if you have a sign like that in your office and you don't honor it, you're a liar. But I digress....

Nobody comes to a doctor's office because they feel fantastic, or because they're happy and everything is perfectly fine. They have a frustration—a problem. There's something wrong. By causing them even more frustration—i.e. being rude to them at the front desk, making them wait in the lobby for an hour or more, and treating them like a number—then you are causing harm. The Hippocratic oath says we are first not to do that.

Having said that, some frustrations are inevitable. We are all extremely busy to start with, and sometimes emergencies come up that cause us to run behind. When you enter a room occupied by a patient who has been kept waiting, one of the most helpful things you can do is confirm their frustration first and foremost. By being proactive about it, you can diffuse the situation. That person is sitting there boiling. Their first reaction when you walk into the room is to let you have it. They want to say, "You know, you made me sit here for an hour! You disrespected me. I have more important things to do than sit here all day." They may not actually say it out loud, but that's what they're thinking.

When I walk into a room and find such a patient, the very first thing I say is, "Mr. Smith, you have been sitting here for a long time. I know how frustrating that is, and I apologize. Let's dive right in and get you moving on with your day."

Guess what they have to do now? They have to agree with you! That is the last thing they wanted to do when you walked in the door. You have completely turned the conversation on its head.

> *If you want to diffuse hard feelings, get the patient to agree with you.*

When you acknowledge your patient's frustration, you change their cortisol level—you lower their stress. This works for more than just their irritation over your being late. If you know the source of their frustration (say, their knee hurts) acknowledge it. If a patient is having surgery or, God forbid, has cancer, it is okay to acknowledge that they're scared. "Cancer does not play fair." Say that to the patient.

"Mrs. Smith, if you're scared and frustrated about this diagnosis and it makes you angry, I want you to know that you are normal. You have every reason to feel that way."

Or, "Mr. Smith, I imagine you are frustrated that this medicine didn't work the way we wanted it to. I am frustrated too. We had high hopes, and it didn't pan out. Let's move on to plan B."

Acknowledging a frustration lessens the effect of it. It disarms people. It's a great way to get a vexing situation back on the right track in a hurry.

ACTION POINTS

1. *Anticipate what a patient's first complaint or frustration may be and acknowledge it. Rarely will you be wrong.*

2. *Confirm to the patient that fear is normal: Fear of the unknown. Fear of pain. Fear of dying. Fear is a normal defense mechanism for patients. Confirm that for them.*

3. *Know that every day will not go as planned. Accept it. Acknowledge when things are not going well and turn your mind toward positive solutions.*

Hello, Old Friend!

Lay this unto your breast: Old friends, like old swords,
still are trusted best.

— JOHN WEBSTER

You know how great it feels when you run into an old friend on the street and they give you the kind of heartfelt greeting that shows you how much they care? You get an instant case of the warm fuzzies. Everybody wants to feel as if they are appreciated. Everybody wants to know that they matter to others. Give your patients the gift of showing them that they matter to you.

Remember, you want to get yourself into your patient's Dunbar's number unit—into the group of people he or she appreciates as friends. If you go into every patient encounter with that intention, you will set yourself up for success. Think about it: you wouldn't run into a dear friend you've known for twenty years and say with a deadpan voice, "Hello, Mr. Smith. I trust you've been well." That is not how you would greet a person you've known for decades, and that is not how you should greet your long-term patients either.

It is okay to walk in and say, "Hey, Bob, how have you been? Gosh, long time no see! What a nice way to start my day—seeing you. Thank you for coming in."

There is nothing wrong with saying that to a patient. In fact it is a good thing. It is the least you can do. This is a person who has come to you for help. They are contributing to your mortgage payment. Acknowledge how great it is to see them. Treat them like an old friend, especially those you've known for years. One of the most wonderful things about medicine is the blessing of getting to know other people on such a personal level. When you stop to think about it, it's actually quite beautiful. Celebrate that with your patients. Because as the old saying goes: the only way to make a friend is to be one.

ACTION POINTS

1. *Greet patients you have known for some time the way you would an old friend.*

2. *Remember that the only way to make a friend is to be one.*

My Patient, the Computer

To effectively communicate, we must realize that we are all different in the way we perceive the world and use this understanding as a guide to our communication with others.

— TONY ROBBINS

I am in love with Siri. There, I said it. Now you know. When I first got my iPhone 4S, I spent an inordinate amount of time talking to Siri, asking her questions, finding out how much she could understand. The problem was that my darling Siri is only a computer, and computers don't really understand anything. They don't have the ability to presume or really know what you're talking about. If you don't believe me, ask your computer to make you a sandwich. I bet you're still hungry afterward. Your computer doesn't know what "sandwich" or "peanut butter" or "jelly" are because it has no reference point it can access until it is given instructions to do so. It has no basis to respond. It can't honor your requests without an actual understanding of what you're talking about.

Your patients are exactly the same way.

That's precisely why I recommend that you communicate with your patients like you do your computer. I know that sounds odd. I know that sounds like it runs counter to everything I've said in this book about treating patients like human beings. But it's true: You have to input data accurately into a computer for it to know what you want it to do. By the same token, you have to input data accurately into your patients before they can follow through. And you have to keep it simple.

"Your diastolic pressure has been consistently high," you say to a patient. But to the vast majority of laypeople, that's just a bunch of mumbo jumbo. They think it sounds important, but they don't know what it means. Does it mean that they are under pressure in their lives? They have not a clue.

Or here's another example. I may say to a patient, "Omega-3 fatty acids are oils that are essential." If you say the words "essential oils" to a massage therapist, an oil rig worker, and a mechanic, you're going to get three different understandings of what that means. When you say "fatty" acids, what are you talking about? Are they going to make the patient fat? Here's another way to approach the subject: "Omega-3 fatty acid is the name of a type of oil or fat that our body cannot produce on its own. Because of that we need some in our diet to give our body what it needs. Certain types of fish and some grains contain it."

So you have to say things in a very simple fashion. You have to break it down and input it in an easily understandable sequence—just as you would when you enter data into a computer. You must lay everything out step by step. "The first step is.... The second step is.... The third step is.... The options are.... The outcome we are seeking is...."

That's how you would key it in to a computer, and that's how you need to key it in to your patients. You can't expect to get the correct output and function from your patients unless you enter the right input and directions. It's just that simple.

ACTION POINTS

1. *Before making a request of or a recommendation to a patient, provide clear, concise information.*

2. *Just because certain words and terms are clear to you, that does not mean they are clear to the patient. Anticipate the level of understanding of the computer — your patient — before inputting data.*

I've Got a Name

I always have trouble remembering three things: faces, names, and — I can't remember what the third thing is.

— FRED ALLEN

Everyone has a name. Every patient has one. I recommend that you use it. Why? People like to hear another person speak their name. It means something to them. It has all their life. And according to research, it's especially important when the person saying their name is their doctor. In fact a 2009 study published in the *BMJ*[9] found that the vast majority of patients under the age of sixty-five said they either didn't mind or they preferred that their doctors called them by their first names.

When you say a name in a sentence, it gives more credence and value to whatever comes after that. For example, "Your blood pressure is high" is not as powerful a statement as, "Diane, your blood pressure is high." Or, "My recommendations are…" is not nearly as meaningful as, "David, this is what I want you to do."

9 B. McKinstry, "Should general practitioners call patients by their first names?" *BMJ* 301 (October 6, 1990): 795, accessed January 9, 2013, doi: http://dx.doi.org/10.1136/bmj.301.6755.795.

Those are different sentences that say essentially the same thing, but the second ones say so much more.

One caveat: I recommend that the first time you meet a patient—especially an older patient—you address them using the title Mr., Ms., or Mrs. Eventually they will invite you to call them by their first name if it makes them comfortable. If not, just continue to call them Mr. Smith or Mrs. Smith, and try to insert that into your sentences as often as you can without sounding ridiculous.

So that's how to address a patient. But how should you introduce yourself? I'm of the opinion that if you have to tell a patient who is sitting in your office that you are Doctor Jones and they are surprised by that, then you have a PR problem. If they don't know who the doctor is by the time you come into the room, you have far bigger issues than can be addressed in this book. Patients know what you do for a living. It seems pretentious to keep reminding them every time you see them, don't you think? Doctors and royalty are the only two groups I know of that cite their occupations before their names. If you want to be lumped in with Prince Charles, go for it. I don't know about you, but I wouldn't necessarily want him providing medical care for me.

Just think about it for a moment. The man who installed your new carpet last week didn't introduce himself to you as Carpet Layer Johnson. The woman who decorated my son's birthday cake last month doesn't call herself Cake Baker Anderson. My wife doesn't go to a salon run by Hairstylist Garcia. People simply don't refer to themselves that way. Medicine is our occupation, and we have good reasons to be proud of that, but I think sometimes we're too proud. Introducing myself to patients as Dr. Koch seems unnecessary. Granted, it establishes a reference point and it sets a respect bar, but respect can also be gained by giving excellent care and establishing rapport and trust with your patients. You don't need to advertise your occupation to them.

So instead of introducing yourself by saying, "I'm Dr. Jones," you can simply say "I'm Angela Jones." You're essentially saying the same thing in those two introductions, but the second one makes you more human. It holds more meaning for your patients. It establishes more of a connection.

You can carry this notion a step further by thinking about the way you introduce and refer to your assistants. They are people too, you know. It's time for a quiz. Which of the following sounds the best to you?

1. My assistant will be in to draw your blood.
2. My assistant, Theo, will be in to draw your blood.
3. Theo, my assistant, will be in to draw your blood.

If you picked the third option, you are correct. Number three is the winner because not only did you use Theo's name, but you also put his name before his job title. You've shown your patient (and, perhaps even more importantly, you've shown Theo) that to you the person is more important than the fact that he's your assistant. When you called him "my assistant" in front of the patient, you sent the signal that it's all about me, Me, ME. But when you called him "Theo, my assistant," he became a human being named Theo who is there to help the patient. That's an important distinction. You said, most importantly, he's a person named Theo, and of second most importance he is your assistant. Remember it the next time you talk about your team members in front of your patients.

ACTION POINTS

1. *A 2009 study published in the BMJ found that the vast majority of patients under the age of sixty-five said they either don't mind or prefer that their doctors call them by their first names.*

2. *Seize every opportunity to include the patient's name in the sentence when conveying information or making recommendations.*

3. *Try introducing yourself by your name and not your occupation.*

4. *When introducing or discussing coworkers, use their names first and foremost, thereby conveying that the people are more important to you than their job titles.*

The Boomerang Effect

By swallowing evil words unsaid,
no one has ever harmed his stomach.

— WINSTON CHURCHILL

You've heard the old adage that goes "if you can't say something nice, don't say anything at all"? Well, it turns out there is a scientific basis for that maxim, and it can have a major impact on doctor-patient relations.

In the 1990s researchers from The Ohio State University at Newark, Purdue University, and Indiana University at Bloomington did a fascinating study[10] on the effects of gossip. In it, participants were shown videos of actors talking about other people. Half of the actors made positive statements and the others made negative statements. Next the research team had the participants rate the personality of each of the speakers in the videos. The actors who described another person negatively were rated negatively, and the actors who described someone positively were viewed to be more positive people.

---

10 John J. Skowronski, Lynda Mae, Matthew T. Crawford, "Spontaneous Trait Transference: Communicators Take on the Qualities They Describe in Others" *The Journal of Personality and Social Psychology* 74, 4.

The results of the study were clear and startling: *even though the listener* knows *the speaker is describing another person's traits, personality, or actions – good or bad – the listener will consistently attribute those traits to the speaker.* The researchers named this phenomenon *spontaneous trait transference;* others have referred to it as *the boomerang effect.* I know it makes no rational sense whatsoever, but it's true. Spontaneous trait transference means that when you gossip with your patients, they will unconsciously assign to you whatever negative traits you are describing. If you want to have that in your pocket as a physician, go for it, but I wouldn't recommend it. It will not win you any points; in fact, as this study shows, you're going to lose points when you do that.

I will also refer you here to the chapter on politics and religion. You never completely know to whom a patient is related or with whom they do business or are otherwise associated. Gossip is dangerous and hurtful, and it isn't practicing medicine. It makes you look bad. If a patient wants you to comment on the downfall of a local business or a person in your community, move the conversation along by changing the subject to positive comments and compliments about something else. You will always be better off.

Here's an example you can probably relate to. When a patient comes in and speaks negatively about another doctor, what do you do? You get nervous. You think, *Wow, am I going to be next on their slam list?* If you are thinking that, then it follows that your patients will think the same if they hear you saying negative things about someone else. As Booker T. Washington once wrote, "One man cannot hold another man down in the ditch without remaining down in the ditch with him."

So it turns out that Mom was right all along. Be nice or keep your lips zipped.

ACTION POINTS

1. *When given the opportunity to gossip to or with a patient, don't. Change the subject with positive comments and compliments.*

2. *Remember: research confirms that speaking negatively about another person casts the speaker in a negative light!*

The Reciprocity Rule

There is one word which may serve as a rule of practice
for all one's life – reciprocity.

— CONFUCIUS

Reciprocity is the foundation of human existence. It is how we have evolved to become the dominant species we are. We have the ability to assist others, to use another person for our benefit, and to help another person for theirs. The *reciprocity rule* states that if you want something from another person, you have to give them something first because doing so triggers an innate desire in them to give something back to you. They owe you.

It has become so expected for indebtedness to come after acceptance of something from another person that the term *much obliged* (obligated) has become synonymous with *thank you*. This is true not only in the United States but in other countries as well. We are taught from the time we are young children to follow this rule, so it has a very powerful influence over us throughout our lifetimes. Remember your mother's constant urging for you to share with your siblings and friends? "Timmy let you play with his blocks. Now you let him play with your fire truck...." This is stuff we all learned in kindergarten, but I don't think most of us realize how to apply it effectively in our adult lives—especially in our lives as healthcare providers.

In his classic book *Influence: The Psychology of Persuasion*, author Robert Cialdini, PhD writes of the rule of reciprocity:

> *One of the reasons reciprocation can be used so effectively as a device for gaining another's compliance is its power. The rule possesses awesome strength, often producing a "yes" response to a request that, except for an existing feeling of indebtedness, would have surely been refused.*

As a medical professional, you want your patients to do you the favor of moving forward in their treatment plans and honoring your requests so they can get better. You want to influence them and persuade them to do things they don't always want to do. To get the ball rolling, you have to give them something first. The gift you give them does not have to be elaborate or expensive to be effective. In fact research shows that recipients can actually show a drop in self-esteem if you overdo it.

You've seen this phenomenon in action. Let's say you have a younger brother who is not as well off in life as you are. If you want to make his self-esteem take a nosedive, give him an extravagantly expensive gift on Christmas morning, and be sure to do it in front of a crowd. It's fun for the whole family…NOT.

When you give someone a gift that makes it obvious you are helping them, it appears that you believe they can't help themselves. Or it looks as if there is an ulterior motive. Giving your patients a dozen roses every time they walk in the door is going to look suspicious. They're going to think you're up to something. Just keep it small and nobody will get hurt.

For example we begin the reciprocity dance in my office with a bowl of chocolate kisses at the front desk. My patients' eyes light up when they see that little bowl of candy. Then we keep the giving going by offering them coffee and water. And everyone who works with me is trained to smile, say "hello," shake hands, and thank patients for coming to our office. Doing so sets the stage for ongoing reciprocity. We've offered them goodwill in tangible and intangible ways. Now they are instinctually stimulated to give us something in return.

We like people who help us, and we help people we like.

Once you've established goodwill by offering the patient something, it's time to make your request and set a timeframe for them to carry it out. Look at these two examples of discussing recommendations with a patient and pick which one you think will be most effective:

"Here is a list of what your blood sugars have been, and here is a list of the recommendations for addressing that. Before our next visit in six months, you should do number one, number two, and number three on that list."

Or...

"Bob, this is what we've done for you here. We've tracked your blood sugars over the last three weeks. Here is the printout of those blood sugar results for you. You can keep that. And here is a printout of the directions you are to follow. You can keep that too. I want you to do numbers one, two, and three on that list before Wednesday."

The first example is unlikely to be followed because (a) you didn't reinforce the fact that you gave the patient something, and (b) the deadline for action is so far in the future it will inevitably go on the back burner. But in the second example, you've called the patient by name. You've given him tangible and intangible things and reminded him of what they are (you've tracked his levels, presented him with the results, and given him a printout of your instructions) and you've established a sense of urgency regarding the timeframe.

Congratulations! You've followed the reciprocity rule to the letter. Now your request is more likely to be honored, and your patient is more likely to have a good outcome.

Everybody wins.

ACTION POINTS

1. *Activate the reciprocity rule with patients first by giving them something of value. This may be an informational brochure, a glass of water, a piece of candy, or even a smile and a compliment.*

2. *When making a recommendation you want the patient to follow, use the patient's name, provide the patient with tangible or intangible value, confirm to the patient that you have provided value, and establish a timeframe (to create a sense of urgency) for following that recommendation.*

Something to Smile About

*When people are smiling, they are most receptive
to almost anything you want to teach them.*

— ALLEN FUNT

Of the forty-seven chapters in this book, chapters one through forty-six should be called "Smile!" Smiling is the quickest, surest, most cost-effective way to grow your fan base of Raving Patients®. When your patients and coworkers see you smiling at them, they interpret that to mean you like them—that you're interested in them. They smile back. And when they smile, the serotonin and dopamine levels in their bodies elevate. In fact the simple act of holding a pencil between your teeth so your mouth forms a smile has the same effect on your own serotonin and dopamine levels. So smiling at your patients is therapeutic. It makes them feel better instantly, without your even having to whip out your prescription pad.

Smiles are consistent across all cultures, and they happen even when there is no intent. You have to teach your child to ride a bike or catch a baseball, but you don't have to teach them to smile. Even a newborn baby will smile when it poops. Smiling is innate. It's instinctual. The first person to arrive at this conclusion scientifically was Guillaume Duchenne, a French anatomist who conducted research in the 1860s into how and why muscles work (this is where the term *Duchenne muscular dystrophy* comes from). Duchenne discovered that a genuine smile begins when emotional information — like spotting a dear friend on the street, feeling the warmth of a hug, or hearing a compliment — enters the brain. That triggers activity throughout the brain, but most notably in the left anterior temporal region, which in turn spurs into action the zygomatic major muscles in the cheeks and the orbicularis oculi around the eyes, causing a genuine smile to spread across the face. People can control their zygomatic major muscles, but only real emotion activates the orbicularis oculi naturally. There's no faking it. That is why it's so easy for us to recognize a phony smile when we see one.

According to recent research, giving someone an authentic smile triggers feelings of altruism in the receiver. In a 2003 French study[11], researchers had an actor walk through a supermarket and smile warmly at half of the random passersby. Within seconds of each smile, another actor standing near the first would drop a bundle of computer discs on the floor. The researchers recorded how many of the passersby stopped to help the second actor pick up the discs. They found that those who had received a smile from the first actor were fifty percent more likely to stop and offer aid to the disc dropper than those who had not received a smile. This study illustrates that receiving a smile — even from a stranger — triggers a positive, cooperative mood. There's really no easier way to put someone in a receptive, healing frame of mind than to smile at them.

Why? Because whenever you give someone a genuine smile, you are activating the power of the reciprocity rule. Remember: when you give another person something, they're obligated to give you something in return. So if you give your patients a smile, they will be more likely to give you the gift of agreeing

---

11 N Guéguen, M-A. De Gail, "The Effect of Smiling on Helping Behavior: Smiling and Good Samaritan Behavior," *Communication Reports* 16, 2 (2003): 133–140.

with your suggestions and following your recommendations for their health.

Therefore smiling at your patients is the best way to set them — and you — up for success.

ACTION POINTS

1. *The act of smiling raises human blood levels of serotonin and dopamine and is therapeutic to patients who smile in natural response to your smile.*

2. *You can activate the reciprocity rule by the simple act of giving smiles to your patients.*

3. *Smile more often and you will feel better more often.*

Emotional Predictions

*...if you can't have empathy and have effective relationships,
then no matter how smart you are,
you are not going to get very far.*

— DANIEL GOLEMAN

In her insightful book *How to Instantly Connect with Anyone*, author Leil Lowndes writes that the trick to relating to others and getting them to relate positively to you in return is to practice the fine art of *emotional prediction*. It's a simple concept, really. Before you begin a dialogue with someone, you must:

- Stop
- Put yourself in the other person's shoes
- Accurately assess what they may be feeling
- Communicate that assessment in a way that shows you care

Predicting your patients' emotions is not too difficult in a medical practice. If someone has to sit in your waiting room for an hour, how do you think they feel? How do you think their emotions are running when you walk in the door? You know. You've probably been there as a patient yourself. They're frustrated.

They're anxious. They're ready to give their doctor a piece of their mind.

But if you walk into that exam room and start the interaction by saying, "Mrs. Smith, you have been sitting here a long time. I know that's frustrating, and I apologize. I'm going to do my best to get you on your way shortly," then you have connected with the patient. Now Mrs. Smith has to agree with you. That is the last thing she expected to do when you walked in the room.

Another example is a patient who has to drive many miles to see you. Check their chart; it probably lists their home city or suburb. Duly noted. "Mr. Smith, thank you for coming. I know you had a long drive all the way from Anytown today, and I appreciate the effort you made to get here." There—you've established that you understand his feelings. You put yourself on his level.

Or this: "Mr. Smith, it's almost lunchtime. You must be hungry. Let's get to these recommendations. Here is what I'd like you to do...." Mr. Smith can't help but agree with you. He's thinking, *Yes, it is almost lunchtime. Yes, I am hungry. Yes, I will do what Dr. Wonderful recommends.*

Moving directly from an agreement connection to a recommendation is key. First you've put yourself on the patient's level and given him a reason to believe you, *then* you've given him your recommendation. You're just keeping the positive ball rolling.

When you accurately predict and express your patients' emotions and then move forward in the conversation, you inject yourself into their psyches in a positive way. You make an important step toward establishing rapport.

Not only can you use this technique to improve patient outcomes, but you can also use it to help you disengage from the unending talker. We've all had the patient who derails our day by continuing to talk nonstop. You'd like to stay and chitchat (or not), but you have to move on. You have a clinic to run. You have a life to lead and a mortgage to pay. You need to have the ability to move away from such a patient in a kind, effective way. Emotional prediction can be your ticket out.

The next time a patient is droning on and on about what's going on in her life yet you have to move on to the next patient, just say exactly that. "Mrs. Smith, I can tell you've got a lot going on in your life, *yet* I have to move on to the next patient." Again, Mrs. Smith has no choice but to agree with you. *Yes, I do have a lot going on in my life,* she thinks. *Yes, I understand that Dr. Wonderful can't stay here all day. Of course she has to move on to the next patient.*

Notice the use of the word *yet* rather than *but*. It is a subtle yet important distinction. *Yet* is a word that connects and relates the proceeding statement to the statement it follows. *But* is a disconnecting word — a separator — that in essence nullifies the proceeding statement. Instead of the word *but* use *yet* in addition to *that, that said*, etc.

Emotional prediction allows you to begin and end your patient interactions with agreement and connection. Your patients will leave your presence feeling good about themselves and about you, and you'll feel better too. That's a major victory for both sides.

ACTION POINTS

1. *Before you begin a dialogue with a patient, put yourself in their shoes and predict how they may be feeling. Communicate and acknowledge your empathy in a way that shows the patient you care.*

2. *When you need to end the conversation and interaction with the unending-talker patient, offer your exit statement directly after an emotional prediction or emotional acknowledgement.*

Body Language

What you do speaks so loudly that I cannot hear what you say.

—RALPH WALDO EMERSON

When you walk into the examining room and you see the patient looking at the ground, slouching, or leaning against a desk looking dejected, it's clear that something is wrong. It's clear that they have a negative perception about something. It's clear that they aren't feeling well.

By the same token, as a healthcare provider, when you walk into the examining room and you're staring at the ground or slouching, or you lean on the desk looking dejected, your patients can see that something is wrong with you, that you have a negative perception about something. That you aren't feeling well.

I don't want to sound like your mother, but chin up, son! Straighten your shoulders. Walk into that room like you're supposed to be there. Open your chest and arms to your patient and nonverbally express to them that you are there on business. You are there to help them feel better.

Even if you don't feel it, fake it until you make it.

Why? Because the reciprocity rule applies to body language too. You get what you give. Be mindful of what you're giving.

For example if you face a patient with empty hands, palms up, held parallel to the floor, that conveys the idea that "I have nothing for you." The last thing you want to convey to them is that you have nothing to offer. Think of your kids. When you ask your young daughter if she stole her brother's cookie, she'll hold her hands palms up and parallel to the floor to show you she has nothing. Don't use that gesture with patients.

Another body language no-no is the shrug. That's what a child does when you ask her if she knows who broke the lamp. She shrugs her shoulders, raises her eyebrows, and gives you that "I don't know" look. Shrugging is just another sign that you have nothing more to offer. It's a signal that you are not going to respond further. It's an indication that you've been put on the spot, that you're holding something in, and that you can't even muster up the energy to vibrate your vocal chords.

Another wishy-washy response is wobbling your head from side to side. This is another sign of uncertainty. If someone asks you where you will be in six months and you bobble your head side to side, that's a sure sign that you don't know. If you're going to move your head in any fashion, make it a nod. When you nod, you acknowledge. And when I say nod, I mean nod up, not down. In other words, start with your chin in the neutral position and have your first nod go up, then back to neutral, then up, and back to neutral. Lifting your chin is an affirmative movement and a positive signal to the patient. It shows that you have confidence and belief in what they said, and that you approve. If a patient tells you he has done well with his blood sugars and he did cardio exercise four out of the last seven days, show your admiration by nodding up while giving him verbal praise. Doing so lends credence to whatever was just said.

When you sit and talk to the patient, are you talking to the patient or to your desk or your iPad? Stop and turn toward the patient. Open your chest and your arms to that person and speak to them as you would to a guest at a party in your home. A good rule to use is to make sure you are pointing your belly button at the patient. This positioning means you are conveying full attention. If your head is turned toward the patient when you speak but your belly button is pointed at your computer, you are not fully engaged with the patient. Think about it. When you're sitting at a party and you're talking with someone, you face them. You don't turn away from them and type on your tablet. When a party guest asks you something, you turn toward them and engage in conversation with them. You turn your entire body so that your belly button points toward the person you are talking with. I don't know why this common courtesy disappears when we converse with our patients, but it does. I see it happen all the time.

If you're sitting in front of a patient and you want them to view you as complacent, sit with your legs extended straight out in front of you and cross them at the ankles. That's what I call "the beach chair" position. That's not the position of someone who is looking forward to acting on whatever his patient is saying. That's the position of someone waiting for the cabana boy to bring another margarita. You're not sitting on a beach. You are a professional sitting in an office full of people who have come to you for help. Point your toes toward the patient and sit with bended knees. You can cross your legs if you like (especially if the patient has her legs crossed, as this is mirroring). That's a sign of a calm attitude. However, don't cross your legs with the ankle on the knee. That creates a crossbow appearance and is less welcoming to the patient.

Lastly there's the great conundrum about what to do with your hands. Use them, but don't point. If you need a lesson in world-class pointing, go to Disney World and ask one of the cast members where the nearest restaurant is. You'll see them point not with one finger, but with their entire hand with all of their fingers held together. They're trained to do it that way because pointing with one finger is considered rude and accusatory. If you need to point a patient down the hallway, do it Disney style with your fingers together and your hand extended in the direction you want the patient to go.

When you want to place emphasis on something you're saying, take a tip from a presidential candidate in a debate. When they want to drive home a point, they don't jab their finger at the other candidate or the moderator because that is considered an aggressive movement. Instead they make a loose fist with their thumb on top of their fingers and they extend that hand in a nonthreatening way to underscore whatever it is they're saying. They anchor the words they are saying with a positive emphasis of body language.

Also, don't raise your hands above your shoulders. That's a scary, menacing motion especially to people who are already stressed, such as the average patient. Just keep your hands between your shoulders and your waist at all times.

Lastly, steepling your hands—touching the fingertips of both hands together—is a great way to place emphasis on a statement. Steepling is well known in literature to convey confidence. When you touch your fingertips together, that indicates unity and agreement. If you want a patient to go along with what you're saying, tap your fingers together while you're talking. If they're explaining something to you and you want to convey that you're listening, bring your fingers together in a steeple. Think of your yoga instructor and her greeting to you. "Namaste," she says. *Namaste* is a greeting that translates to "my spirit honors yours." With her hands in the steeple position and a kind acknowledgement she conveys her respect to you.

You can honor your patients in the same fashion. This gesture indicates thoughtfulness and attention. Patients who perceive their doctor as thoughtful, attentive, and honorable are going to be happier patients, which, as we now know, makes us (and our malpractice insurers) happier too.

ACTION POINTS

1. *Enter each room with the body language of a person who is meant to be there to make a positive difference in someone else's life.*

2. *Point your belly button (not just your head) at the person to whom you are speaking.*

3. *Use your hands for emphasis and for anchoring important points in your conversation. One way to do this is by steepling your fingers together to indicate unity and agreement. Remember the namaste greeting of honor and use a kind nod or steepled hands to convey that you understand.*

4. *Use nods of the head to acknowledge positives from your patient. Nod upward: start with your head in the neutral position and nod up and back to neutral, conveying uplifting confirmation of what the patient said.*

5. *Mirror your patient's body position during a conversation to establish a subconscious connection with them.*

Healing Vocabulary

The words of truth are simple.

— AESCHYLUS

As healthcare providers our words can either inspire our patients to move forward toward wellness or stop them in their tracks. That's why it's critically important to spend time developing a cache of motivational words and phrases you can draw upon at will, and use them to strengthen and motivate your patients every day.

In his book *Unstoppable Confidence*, author Kent Sayre lists several words he refers to as "confidence killers" and suggests readers eliminate them from their vocabularies in order to become more self-assured. I agree, especially when it comes to those of us working in healthcare. Sayre's confidence-killing words — *try*, *hope*, and *but* — really have no place in your interactions with patients.

Try

"Do or do not. There is no try," said Yoda in *Star Wars: The Empire Strikes Back*. That was sage advice for Luke Skywalker, and it is sage advice for you as well. *Try* is a weak, watered-down, wishy-washy half word. It means that maybe you will, maybe you won't.

Try does not inspire confidence that there will be success—heck, it doesn't even necessarily mean there's going to be much effort.

When you make a recommendation to a patient and they say, "I'll try," how confident are you that they will succeed? Not very. And when you say to a patient, "I want you to try to get some exercise each week," how inspired do you think they're going to be by that? Again, not very.

Therefore never suggest to your patients that they try to follow your recommendations. Be assertive. Tell them that you *want* them to follow your recommendations—that you *expect* them to do it. Instead of "I want you to try to get some exercise," say, "I want you to do cardio exercise four out of seven days each week." There's nothing wishy-washy about that.

And if they say in response, "OK, I'll try," stop them right there and remind them that when it comes to their health, there is no try—only do.

Trust me, when you eliminate the word *try* from your and your patients' vocabularies, the Force will be with you and with them. Go ahead. Insert your Star Wars nerd jokes about me here. It's OK. I'm laughing too. Just remember: Do or do not. There is no try.

Hope

"I hope you'll get some exercise next week, Mrs. Smith," you say.

Well, isn't that nice, Mrs. Smith thinks. *Dr. Wonderful hopes I'll exercise. He can hope all he wants, but I'm not hauling my fanny up off the couch.*

Hoping that something will happen is no more effective than tossing coins into a fountain. *Hope* is not an action word. It is a wish and nothing more. Don't misunderstand. I am not saying you shouldn't have high hopes for your patients—of course you should be hopeful and of course you should communicate that. I'm sure your intentions are good. It's just that simply telling your patients that you hope they'll follow your recommendations is not necessarily going to elicit action.

Statements like "I hope this helps," "I hope this does the trick," or "I hope we can get this to improve" do not command change. You have only inferred your wish and that's it. No action, no time urgency. No positive expectation.

Instead of saying, "I hope you will take this medicine every single day until it's gone," say, "David, it is important that you take this medicine every single day until it's gone." The latter is an action sentence, and it is much more likely to inspire compliance than the first.

But

When I was young, I learned that the word *but* is only an acronym for **b**ehold the **u**nderlying **t**ruth. What an accurate assessment. When you use the word *but* in a sentence, you are contradicting your own point. You are negating everything you said before "but." Here, for example, is my personal favorite *but* sentence:

"I'm not prejudiced, BUT...."

Behold, the **u**nderlying **t**ruth is that you *are* prejudiced. When someone says something like that, they are talking nonsense.

When a patient tells me, "I really want to lose weight BUT I don't have time to exercise," I disregard everything they said before "but." It doesn't mean a thing. It's as if a giant tree just fell across the road in the middle of that sentence.

More often than not the word *but* is placed where the period at the end of the sentence should be. You will stop contradicting yourself when you stop using that word followed by a statement of why what you said before it was false. Instead say, "I'm not prejudiced." "I really want to lose weight." PERIOD. End of positive statement.

No buts about it — you must eliminate *but* from your vocabulary, and don't let your patients get away with using it either.

And while we're on the subject of words to eliminate, let's talk about immature speech patterns. I am all for building rapport with patients, but you still have to maintain proper English. I am stunned by some of the things I've heard come out of doctors' mouths of late.

"Dude, seriously? You need to take your meds."

"I'm not harshing on you, man, but you really need to drop some pounds. I'm telling you."

"So I'm like recommending that you like have this test? And then we'll like hook up again next week and like discuss the results? And we'll like go from there. OK?"

OMG! Those kinds of immature speech patterns need a doctor! Overcome them immediately. The professionalism you save may be your own.

Sick Speak Versus Power Words

Should-a, would-a, could-a — anything that ends in -ould means uncertainty. Should, would, and could signify no commitment whatsoever. They are not action words. If they do elicit a response, it's negative.

Avoid those sick-speak words. Instead use power words like:

- absolutely
- certainly
- definitely
- undoubtedly
- obviously
- will
- know

Absolutely you will. You definitely will. You certainly can. You obviously have. You undoubtedly have the ability to. Without a doubt I know that you can. Those are all modal operators — phrases that say essentially the same thing as *should, could* and *would* except that they are affirmative and they elicit action. When you use modal operators in your speech, you erase doubt.

"You should feel better after taking this medication," you say to Mrs. Smith.

Yes, I should, she thinks, *but that doesn't mean I will.*

"You should feel better" is not nearly as motivating and powerful as, "Mrs. Smith, there's absolutely no doubt in my mind that you will feel better when you use this medication."

Wow. That's a powerful, affirming sentence. There's nothing wrong with saying that to a patient. When you say you have no doubt about her treatment plan, Mrs. Smith's confidence level is going to go up. And that will encourage her to take her meds, which will lead to a good outcome...and another Raving Patient.

ACTION POINTS

1. *Cleanse your vocabulary of confidence-killing words like* try, hope, *and* but. *Instead use assertive words that command action* (can, will, expect, now).

2. *The word* but *often negates the meaning of the words or thoughts that come before it in the sentence. End your statement where you would have previously used the word* but *and note the positive effect and power it has on the meaning you want to convey.*

3. *Utilize power words such as* absolutely, certainly, definitely, will, *and* can *to instill confidence in the patient about your recommendations.*

The Franklin Effect

He that has once done you a kindness will be more ready to do you another than he whom you yourself have obliged.

— BEN FRANKLIN

I wrote in an earlier chapter that if you want to make a friend, first you must be one. But there's an interesting twist to that, and it's described in the Ben Franklin quote above. It's true—when someone does a favor for you, their warm feelings for you increase and they are more willing to cooperate with you in the future. Here's the backstory to Franklin's quote:

As legend has it, Franklin needed an agreement from an adversary in the House of Representatives on some legislation he was putting forth, but the congressman had always been indifferent to Franklin in the past. Knowing that the congressman was a rare-book collector, and having heard that he had an exceedingly scarce book in his collection, Franklin wrote a note asking the congressman if he could borrow that particular book for a few days. The congressman sent the book over. Franklin followed through exactly as he said he would. He returned the book on schedule along with a note thanking the congressman for his kind generosity in loaning it to him.

And lo and behold, soon after Franklin's expression of gratitude for the favor of allowing him to enjoy such a rare book,
the congressman decided to change his position and support
Franklin's legislation. It was like magic. Franklin described it
this way:

> *When we next met in the House, he spoke to me (which he had
> never done before), and with great civility; and he ever after mani-
> fested a readiness to serve me on all occasions, so that we became
> great friends, and our friendship continued to his death.*[12]

And that's the Franklin effect: when somebody does you a
favor—and it doesn't have to be a big one—they think of you as
more likeable. They are more likely to do even more favors for
you going forward.

Modern research has validated this phenomenon, most notably Jecker and Landy's 1969 study entitled "Liking a Person
as a Function of Doing Him a Favour." In it a group of participants were pitted against one another in a knowledge contest,
and the winners were rewarded with money. Next a researcher
asked some of the winners to do him the favor of returning their
cash prize, explaining that he had used his own personal money
for the study and he was running low on funds. The other winners were not approached and were allowed to keep their money.
The scientists then surveyed all the participants to see how much
they liked the researcher. In accordance with the Franklin effect,
the participants who had done the researcher the favor of returning the money ranked him higher on the likeability scale than
those who had not been asked.

---

12 "The Autobiography of Benjamin Franklin, Chapter Nine," Archiving Early
America, accessed January 15, 2013, www.earlyamerica.com/lives/franklin/
chapt9/.

Jecker and Landy wrote:

It is generally assumed that a person performs favors for people whom he likes; in fact, doing a favor for someone is itself often an expression of esteem. Is it possible, however, that a person comes to like those people for whom he performs favors? We contend that it is. Under certain circumstances, when an individual performs a favor for another person, his liking for that person will increase.[13]

Therefore ask each of your patients to do you a favor. They'll like you more afterward, and their willingness to do even more favors for you in the future will increase. You don't have to ask them to do anything earth-shattering. Keep it simple.

For example ask an older, sedentary patient to do you the favor of walking to the end of their block and back today, and then request that they call and leave a message letting you know they did it and how it went. Or ask a patient to do you the favor of calling and leaving a message with his blood pressure reading later that night. The walk and the blood pressure may not actually matter to you at all, but getting those patients to do you the favor does matter. Simply establish the precedent of having your patient do one little favor for you and they will be more likely to honor your requests when it really counts.

ACTION POINTS

1. *Utilize the Franklin effect by first asking your patient to do you a very small favor. After obliging your first simple request, they will be more likely to honor and follow through on your larger, more meaningful recommendations in the future.*

---

13 Jon Jecker, David Landy, "Liking a Person as a Function of Doing Him a Favour," *Human Relations* 22, 4 (1969): 371–378.

Anchoring

Every closed eye is not sleeping,
and every open eye is not seeing.

— BILL COSBY

If you have ever haggled over the price of a car at a dealership, you have experienced the effect of anchoring. *Anchoring* is the human propensity to rely too much on the first bit of information we receive when making a decision. When you walk up to a car on the lot, the first piece of information you receive about it is the price — the giant numbers the dealer put on the windshield. That price is your set point. They color all subsequent judgments you will make as the negotiations go forward.

When dealers stick those numbers on the car, they know they probably will not sell the car for that amount. Those numbers are there only to establish an anchor in the potential buyer's mind: *this is the point where the negotiations will begin.* Even when the buyer believes he knows what the car is actually worth, he will still be unduly influenced by the anchor the dealer has planted in his psyche.

In a 1974 study entitled "Judgment under Uncertainty: Heuristics and Biases,"[14] researchers Amos Tversky and Daniel Kahneman tested the theory of anchoring. In one experiment they asked study participants to calculate quickly in their heads the product of the numbers one through eight using these formulas:

$$1 \times 2 \times 3 \times 4 \times 5 \times 6 \times 7 \times 8$$

$$8 \times 7 \times 6 \times 5 \times 4 \times 3 \times 2 \times 1$$

Those are the same numbers only reversed. In the first set of numbers, the anchor is the number one because it is the first thing you see. In the second the anchor is the number eight. When participants tried to solve the problem quickly in their heads using the first set with one as the anchor, the average calculation was 512. But when they tried to solve the problem using the second formula with an anchor of eight, the average guess was much higher: 2,250.[15] The lower the anchor, the lower the estimate and vice versa.

The study showed that anchoring is innate and universal. We anchor to the first thing we see, and we adjust from there. This goes back to what Malcolm Gladwell wrote in *Blink*. Judgments are established within the first ten seconds.

Put this in the context of a medical office. A new patient shows up for an appointment, and you can see she is disheveled in her appearance. Her slacks are dirty, her hair is mussed, her fingernails are chipped and grimy, and her makeup is smudged. That's your anchor. And what conclusion do you draw from that? That the woman doesn't take care of herself? That she doesn't practice good hygiene? You don't know for sure, but you're anchoring with that negative perception. The truth is she had to change a

---

14 Amos Tversky; Daniel Kahneman, "Judgment under Uncertainty: Heuristics and Biases," *Science* 185, 4157. (September 27, 1974): 1124–1131, accessed January 15, 2013, www.hss.caltech.edu/~camerer/Ec101/JudgementUncertainty.pdf.
15 The correct answer is 40,320.

flat tire on the way to your office and there wasn't enough time for her to go home, freshen up, and still make her appointment with you. It's not that she is a sloppy person; it's that she respected your time so much she didn't want to be late for her meeting with you.

It's instinctive for us to anchor to our first judgment. You must be ever mindful of your natural propensity toward anchoring and work hard to remind yourself that your anchor may not always be correct. Also know that your patients are going to anchor as well. They are going to anchor to your staff's actions, to your body language, to the décor in the lobby. Let them anchor to something positive. Set the bar high. Let them anchor to a smile, a welcoming office, and a warm greeting.

Give your patients the benefit of the doubt and they'll probably do the same for you.

ACTION POINTS

1. *Start each patient interaction with a mental anchor of positive improvement and the expectation of educating the patient about how they can and will improve.*

2. *Set your own anchor point with the patient within the first ten seconds of your visit by exuding a positive, welcoming demeanor.*

The Three Hundred Rule

Late in his career, [baseball legend Joe] DiMaggio was asked why he hustled on a play that meant little in a game that had little bearing on the Yankee's fate that year. "Because there is always some kid who may be seeing me for the first time," DiMaggio explained. "I owe him my best."

— FROM WHAT MADE DIMAGGIO A GREAT PLAYER
BY DENNIS GAFFNEY

The other night on television, I watched Aerosmith and Steven Tyler perform the classic rock anthem "Walk This Way." It was a marvel. That song sounded just as great as it did the first time I heard it back when I was a kid. I thought, *I wonder how many times Steven Tyler has sung that song over the years? Probably a million, yet he still pours his heart and soul into it every time.*

But what if one night Steven Tyler decided he'd had enough? What if he just walked out onto the stage at Madison Square Garden wearing baggy sweatpants and a Fruit-of-the-Loom T-shirt and told the thousands of screaming fans who had paid good money to attend his concert, "Look, this is probably the billionth time I've had to sing this stupid song. I'm bored as hell doing this. Let's just get this over with, OK?"

But that never happens. Instead Tyler puts his glittery scarves on the microphone stand, hits the stage, dances around like a wild man, and sings that same song over and over, night after night. And he sings it with passion because he knows there are people out there paying to hear him express it that way. Those concert-goers want to gain a feeling from what he's saying. They expect it. No, they *deserve* it.

Your patients are no different at all except the stakes are higher. They are relying on you for so much more.

If you expect to stay popular and be watched and listened to for decades like Steven Tyler, you have to walk the talk. You have to mean what you say and say what you mean, and do it the right way every single day.

That's what the three hundred rule is all about. Believe me, I understand how it is. You've explained the benefits of exercise and lower cholesterol three hundred times this month alone, and even though it's redundant and unending and tedious and tiresome to you, and now you have to walk into a room and say it for the three hundred and first time, you have to *stop and remember this may be the first time this patient has ever heard it.* You need to explain those benefits to this patient with passion. You need to express them with meaning. You need to say them with emphasis. Even though every fiber of your being is telling you just to walk in that room, roll your eyes, and say, "Blah, blah, blah, exercise, blah, blah, blah, lower cholesterol, blah, blah, blah," you must summon the strength to overcome that temptation and address your patient in an expressive, enthusiastic, and compassionate way.

Do Steven Tyler proud. Give it everything you've got every single time, for every single patient. Set a great example for your patients and show them how to "walk this way."

ACTION POINTS

1. *Even though you may have had the same conversation and made the same recommendations three hundred times, say it as if it were the first time. It may be the first time the patient has ever heard it. Say it with passion and enthusiasm every time.*

Practice Unselfishness

We cannot hold the torch to light another's path
without brightening our own.

— BEN SWEETLAND

I was honored one year to be a member of the admissions committee at a Big Ten university medical school. For months we pored over one admission essay after another from fresh-faced young people who each said it was their dream to become a doctor because they wanted to help people. Never once did I read an essay that said the applicant was going into medicine for the money.

But lately it seems that many of us have forgotten what we wrote in our own admission essays. When you have in the back of your mind an ulterior motive such as money, recognition, or fame, your practice becomes tainted by that. Now, I'm not too clueless to know that you have a mortgage to pay and kids to send through college. This is a business, after all. But either you can choose to charge through it tediously with the tangible benefits as your primary goal or you can enjoy it for the beautiful, unique intangibles you can't find in any other field.

You receive your greatest gifts only when you stop worrying about what you will receive.

Do you find yourself asking the business office if a patient has insurance before you walk into the exam room? Do you first inquire whether or not a patient pays your bills before you decide which tests you're going to run or which questions you're going to answer? Don't you think the way you practice medicine is tainted if you're doing that?

I think it is.

Oftentimes I see colleagues go on medical mission trips to foreign countries, yet our free clinics on the east side of our own city sit empty because they can't find enough doctors to volunteer. It always puzzles me that these colleagues are able to foot the bill to travel to and practice in an exotic locale for a week but they can't drive five blocks down the street to help their neighbors in need. Helping local folks is easier. It costs less money. You can probably help just as many people if not more. But there is one big difference between serving in the free clinic and serving in an exotic place: public gratification versus personal gratification. Working at the free clinic on the east side is not sexy. You're not going to hear a lot of applause. It doesn't make for great slideshows when you return home. When you're at the free clinic, you're not sending out tweets from Botswana as evidence of how important and generous you are.

Always examine your motives carefully. Are they transparent and pure or are they ulterior?

Case in point: A cancer center in my community solicited donations from local businesses for a benefit they had coming up. A cosmetic physician generously donated a wrinkle treatment and spa package for inclusion in the silent auction. But when he discovered that another cosmetic surgeon had also donated a package, he withdrew his contribution. So obviously it wasn't about cancer at all, was it? He wasn't interested in helping people. He was solely interested in self-promotion. I can't imagine anybody reading this paragraph and not thinking, *Ick.* It was one of the most brazenly arrogant things I have ever witnessed in my life.

That's what wrongheaded attachments to tangible rewards can do to a person. They turn you into a selfish isolate. Attachments like that drag you down from behind. When you can untangle yourself from them once and for all, the real benefits of practicing medicine will grow and grow. You'll feel free. You'll sleep well at night. Ken Blanchard wrote, "People with humility don't think less of themselves; they just think of themselves less." In order to be happy in this business, that is what we must strive for. Humility and unselfishness are two of the greatest, most endearing attributes you can express as a doctor. Your patients will appreciate knowing that you are human—that you're willing to give of yourself.

I'd like to offer one final example of unselfishness from a source you probably wouldn't expect: a huge pharmaceutical corporation. In our collective mind, pharmaceutical companies are money-hungry Death Stars (there's the Star Wars nerd again). They are generally considered the dark side of this business. But in the mid-1980s, the pharma giant Merck & Co. began developing a drug named ivermectin to treat onchocerciasis, also known as river blindness. Onchocerciasis is a parasitic disease transmitted by a black-fly bite that leads to severe rashes and blindness, among other unfortunate things. It was (and still is) primarily a disease of developing countries; unfortunately the people who needed the drug the most were those who could never afford to pay for it.

Merck & Co. developed ivermectin anyway. They were on top of something big, and they knew the drug could help millions of people. In 1987 it cleared the final FDA trials and the company began giving it away for free to anyone who needed it. To date more than three hundred million tablets have been donated. No fanfare, no parade, just help. That's an example of giving anonymously without any expectation of return. Merck & Co. didn't have to develop ivermectin. They didn't gain anything tangible from it. In fact it was an absolute money loser for them, but it was a winner for humanity.

The more you do things like that, the better you will be — and the better we will all be.

We are healthcare providers, not health *bill and collect money* providers. Our days (and, for many of us, our nights) are spent treating people with problems. We've all taken call. We've all stayed up late. We've all been dog tired when the last patient of the day showed up fifteen minutes past their appointment. We've all needed to get home and drive our daughter to dance class only to have a last-minute emergency prevent us from leaving the office. We've all treated patients even though we knew there was little likelihood of getting paid. I've never met a homeless doctor, but I have met a few who valued money over the value of caring for another human being.

Caring. That's what it means to be a doctor. That's part of the business of helping people when they need it the most — and there are few things in life that hold greater personal reward than that. Let that be your guidepost each day. If you do I promise that, when all is said and done, you will never regret your career choice.

ACTION POINTS

1. *Donate your time, money, and/or knowledge anonymously.*

2. *Help where help is needed most, not where you gain the most personal notoriety. When you do that you will never wonder if your investment was worth it.*

Get Used To Being Uncomfortable

Comfort zones are most often expanded through discomfort.

— PETER MCWILLIAMS

If all healthcare providers in the world always knew exactly the right things to say to their patients, if every single patient interaction were completely effortless and ideal, there would be no need for me to write this book and there would be no need for you to pick it up. But the practice of medicine isn't a faultlessly choreographed waltz of absolute perfection. It is the polar opposite of that because whenever people are involved, someone's going to get their toes stepped on. There are going to be some awkward, sloppy, uncomfortable moments.

Ah, people. You gotta love 'em. As my father used to say, "Everybody's different. It doesn't mean they're wrong, it just means they're different." And believe me, each and every one of those "differents" will make their way into your office at some point. There are abrasive people in this world. There are people who don't have the ability to think as quickly as others. There are folks who yell when they talk and others whose speech is inaudible, like a dog whistle. There are some who mumble and there are some who stutter. There are people who move at the speed of pond fungus and others who are so fidgety they're bouncing off the walls.

When you encounter these kinds of challenging people in your practice, you will have to be the one to make the appropriate adjustments. Because here's a news flash: when you're a healthcare provider, you are there for the patient's comfort. They are not there for yours. If a patient has hemorrhoids and can't sit, then talk to her while she's walking around the room if it makes her feel better. To insist that a patient sits in a certain area or in a certain way is not helpful to them. That's not for their comfort; it's for yours.

When patients say something that you're not particularly interested in or that you're uncomfortable with (for example if you're a cosmetic surgeon and they're telling you about their hemorrhoids), it's because that story means something to them. Listen to them even if it's boring, and then efficiently move the conversation forward. Acknowledge what they're saying. I'm not suggesting you have to treat those hemorrhoids. I'm simply suggesting they wouldn't have brought it up if it weren't important to them. You can handle a little discomfort if that's what it takes to get your job done. It's OK. It's to be expected.

When I think of discomfort, I am reminded of the first lunar landing back in 1969. The Apollo 11 command module that carried the astronauts on that mission was the opposite of spacious. It wasn't luxurious and it certainly wasn't comfortable, but it was efficient. It got the job done. It changed history. The astronauts riding in that module knew they had to get used to being uncomfortable because they had a job to do: get to the moon and back. That cramped, little module was the only way.

That's what I mean when I say it's OK to be uncomfortable. Just knowing that in and of itself is a reassurance. When you're uncomfortable with something or someone, recognize it within yourself but don't let it show. Don't squint or grimace. Don't turn away. It's your job to offer comfort, not to be uncomfortable in front of the patient. Do whatever it takes to communicate effectively and put them at ease. And remember this excerpt from one of my favorite books by John Maxwell:

...make decisions based on what works best and what is right rather than what may be commonly accepted. Know this, in your early years you won't be as wrong as people think you are. In your later years you won't be as right as people think you are. And all through the years, you will be better than you thought you could be.[16]

ACTION POINTS

1. *Anticipate and accept that as a healthcare provider, you will be in uncomfortable situations at times. Keep your discomfort to yourself and provide comfort to the patient. The Apollo 11 rocket capsule wasn't comfortable. It was efficient and effective, and it changed human history.*

---

16 John C. Maxell, *How Successful People Think: Change Your Thinking, Change Your Life* (New York: Center Street, 2009), 91.

Attitude of Gratitude

Gratitude is the sign of noble souls.

— AESOP

Gratitude is a basic tenet of human (and, for that matter, non-human) interaction. Ask your dog if he's happy when you give him a treat. See his tail wag? He's grateful, believe me. Ask your patient if she's happy when you approach her with kindness and respect. You can be sure she's grateful for that. What are you grateful for? Are you giving voice to that gratitude?

Study after study shows that expressing gratitude improves your health and well-being, your attitude going forward, your relationships with others, and your life in general. One such study from 2003 by Emmons and McCullough[17] showed that people who kept a daily gratitude journal reported fewer health complaints, exercised more, slept better, and were more satisfied with their lives than those who kept a daily journal filled with neutral or negative entries. When you express your appreciation for something, you stay thankful — you feel great-full, or full of

17 R.A. Emmons, M.E. McCullough, "Counting blessings versus burdens: An experimental investigation of gratitude and subjective well being in daily life," *Journal of Personality and Social Psychology* 84 (2003): 377–89.

greatness. You just feel better, and it makes the person to whom you're expressing it feel better too.

In a 2011 *New York Times* article called "A Serving of Gratitude May Save the Day," Michael E. McCullough of the University of Miami said:

> *More than any other emotion, gratitude is the emotion of friend-ship. It is part of a psychological system that causes people to raise their estimates of how much value they hold in the eyes of another person. Gratitude is what happens when someone does something that causes you to realize that you matter more to that person than you thought you did.*[18]

If you want to be a better, friendlier, more successful health-care provider, be grateful and *show* it. As William Arthur Ward once said, "Feeling gratitude and not expressing it is like wrap-ping a present and not giving it." When your patients follow your recommendations or otherwise do something good, they've helped you do your job better and they've helped you pay your mortgage. Always remember that your patients are your custom-ers. If there are no patients, there are no collections. Healthcare is a business. Admittedly we have to run our business a bit dif-ferently from the average corporation, but they are businesses nonetheless. Be grateful for the customers who patronize your healthcare business. Let them know that you notice their efforts and that you are thankful.

When I talk to a parent before and after their child's surgery, I always say, "Thank you for trusting me with the most important person in your life. That's quite an honor, and it that means a lot to me." When I say that to people, I can see the effect those words have on them. It comforts them, strengthens them, and softens

---

18 John Tierney, "A Serving of Gratitude May Save the Day," *The New York Times*, November 21, 2011, accessed January 18, 2013, http://www.nytimes.com/2011/11/22/science/a-serving-of-gratitude-brings-healthy-dividends.html.

their hearts all at the same time. They really *are* trusting me—a lot. They deserve my thanks.

When the spouse or partner of one of your patients is being supportive—perhaps they're helping the patient to quit smoking, or take their medication, or lose weight—always express your gratitude to them. Say, "Mrs. Smith, thank you so much for helping me with Bob's care. I appreciate your efforts. We're going to get to this goal. Together we will." That person is helping you do your job. Why not thank them for that?

And when a patient calls with a question about their care—maybe they want clarification on the dosage of a medication, or they have concerns about a possible allergic reaction—thank them for calling, and thank them for their question. You are already on the phone and you have to say something. Make it a positive experience for both of you.

"But Brent," you say, "that will only encourage them to call more often!" On the contrary, people do not want to be a bother to someone they like. If you want to be a doctor but do not want to answer questions, please look into other occupational options. Those patients with questions are doing your job for you. Your job is to avoid allergic reactions, figure out how medications work for each patient, make sure the dosage is correct, and understand how the patient is feeling. When a patient calls in to tell you those things, they're helping. We tend to forget that.

I'm not saying to reward the patient who calls twenty times in five days. I've been there. It happens, but it's rare. What I am saying is that most people are reasonable. If you greet them with, "Thank you for calling. That's a fantastic question. Let's get to the bottom of this together," you're going to come out ahead. Look, you're going to have to take the call anyway. You can either be an ass or be a person of gratitude.

Guess which one gets more referrals?

Your job is to care for sick people. Here's a pearl for you: caring for sick people means answering questions when people are sick. Patients aren't scared only between the hours of 8:00 a.m. and 4:00 p.m. Monday through Friday. Pain doesn't stop just because it's the weekend. Your job continues.

Acknowledge your patients' participation in their own care, and thank them for it. Your kindness will be rewarded because gratitude is one of the few healthy things in life that is contagious (so are smiles). Be thankful for your patients and they will be thankful right back.

Gratitude is not only the *right* thing, it is a *profitable* thing. The next time you fly on a commercial airline or go to Disney World, count how many times you hear "thank you" and other expressions of gratitude. "Thank you for flying the friendly skies." "Thank you for your attention." "Thank you for your patience." Heck, they even thank you for not smoking and for not lighting an incendiary device on a commercial airliner! Why? Because being thanked makes customers happy. Customers equal sales. Happy customers return, and business thrives. We are in business too—the healthcare business. Make it profitable for everyone involved. Say "thank you" at every opportunity and your business will thrive.

Another important, profitable, and underestimated group when it comes to gratitude is your own staff and coworkers. Thank your employees. Thank your team members. You may have had a manager or senior staff member who was of the "that is what the employees are there for" mindset. "Why thank *them*? The employees should thank me for giving them a job." How did it make you feel about them? Not exactly someone you want to go the extra mile for. It is very easy to say, "Thanks! I know it's just part of your job, but I appreciate your enthusiasm and the pride you take in your work. It helps everyone." Praise like that goes a long way toward motivating your team members. When you need them most, they will be more likely to help because they know their help is appreciated.

ACTION POINTS

1. *Each day, take note of what you are grateful for. Write it down or tell someone else.*

2. *Express your appreciation and say "thank you" to your patients. They are giving you the gift of trust. They are also paying your salary.*

3. *Show your gratitude to your team members with praise for a job well done.*

You've Got the Touch

Too often we underestimate the power of a touch, a smile,
a kind word, a listening ear, an honest compliment, or the
smallest act of caring, all of which have the potential to turn a
life around.

— LEO BUSCAGLIA

Human touch is a powerful thing — and a fascinating research topic. There have been a number of studies showing that lightly touching another person's upper arm for only an instant when you make a request increases their compliance. In a widely cited study from 1977,[19] researchers had an actor approach people in a telephone booth (remember those?) and ask, "Excuse me, did I leave a dime in the coin return?" In half the cases, the actor momentarily touched the person lightly on the upper arm when he asked the question; in the other half of the cases, there was no touch. The people who were touched helped the actor look for the dime 20 percent more often than did the people who were not touched.

---

19 C.L. Klienke, "Compliance to requests made by gazing and touching experimenters in field settings," *Journal of Experimental Social Psychology* 13, 3 (1977): 218–223.

In a similar study from 1980,[20] researchers approached people on the street and asked them to sign a petition. When making the request, the researchers gently touched the upper arms of half of the people; the others were not touched. Of those who were not touched, 55 percent agreed to sign the petition. Of those who were touched, 81 percent complied.

In a 2003 study,[21] researcher Nicolas Guéguen wrote, "Strangers who are touched lightly on the upper arm helped pick up an object [dropped on the street] ninety percent of the time as opposed to sixty percent when they were not touched."

And then there was this fascinating study from 2006[22] in which researchers investigated the power of emotional communication through touch. Participants were lightly touched on the arm by an actor whom they could not see, and they were asked to identify which emotion the actor was attempting to convey through that touch. The emotions included gratitude, sympathy, fear, love, disgust, and anger. The participants were able to correctly identify the emotion up to 83 percent of the time. For the sake of context, those are essentially the same results we get when we are able to see the other person.

In study after study—whether the technique was used by waitstaff in a restaurant, supermarket taste testers, charity workers, or political candidates wanting to leave a sign in a yard—when upper-arm touch was involved, response went up and compliance improved. The bottom line is that people are more likely to be agreeable after they've been touched gently on the upper arm.

You can utilize this technique in your conversations with patients, friends, family members, and even your staff to improve

20 F.N. Willis Jr., H.K. Hamm, "The use of interpersonal touch in securing compliance," *Journal of Nonverbal Behavior* 5, 1 (1980): 49–55.

21 N. Guéguen, J. Fischer-Lokou, "Tactile contact and spontaneous help: and evaluation in a natural setting," *Journal of Social Psychology* 143, 6 (December 2003): 785–7.

22 M.J. Hertenstein, D. Keltner, B. App, B.A. Bulleit, A.R. Jaskolka, "Touch communicates distinct emotions," *Emotion*, 6, 3 (August 2006): 528–33.

efficiency in the clinic environment. If you want a patient to follow through on their physical therapy, lightly tap them on the upper arm while you say, "When you do your physical therapy, it will help strengthen and increase flexibility in your knee and help you feel fantastic after surgery."

I'm sure you can think of a thousand different scenarios in which you can test this theory. So get busy with that, but before you start I want to be sure to include the inevitable disclaimer: While I do advocate that you touch your patients, let me be very clear. This is platonic touch on the upper arm I'm talking about. Don't for a second gather any absurd notion that I'm advocating inappropriate touching. That's against the law, and it's yucky.

Also, being touched can have quite different meanings to different people depending upon the situation, the recipient's culture, and the genders of those involved. Generally speaking, the upper arm is regarded as the safest place to touch someone you don't know, but you also have to use some common sense and intuition.

The bottom line is that you're a medical professional. Act professionally at all times and you should be just fine using this incredibly compelling technique.

ACTION POINTS

1. *When seeking compliance with your recommendations, consider using an inconspicuous touch on the patient's upper arm.*

2. *Remember that in study after study — whether the technique was used by waitstaff in a restaurant, supermarket taste testers, charity workers, or political candidates wanting to leave a sign in a yard — when upper-arm touch was involved, response went up and compliance improved.*

Pessimism Is a Treatable Disease

A pessimist is never disappointed.

— JACK CLEARY

According to Encarta Dictionary, pessimism is "the tendency to see only the negative or worst aspects of all things, and to expect only bad or unpleasant things to happen." Synonyms for pessimism include *cynicism, sadness, dejection, distrust, gloom, grief, melancholy,* and *unhappiness.* Those play no role whatsoever in helping patients improve their medical condition, yet pessimism is epidemic today.

But that doesn't mean that the pessimistic patient is doomed forever. This is a disease that can be treated. Step number one in the treatment plan is to get the patient to face the truth. If you're treating a pessimistic patient, they will say things like:

"I can't lose that much weight. There is no way."

"I can't get my sugars under control."

"It hurts too much to exercise, and I don't have the time."

In their minds they're being realistic. They're being pragmatic. But there is a fine line between pragmatism and pessimism, and that line can be stepped over. Ask yourself and the patient if their view is realistic. Is what they are saying reasonable? Sometimes it is. Poor health hurts. But cynicism weakens the heart, body, mind, and soul even further. Negativity destroys relationships. Pessimism breaks down communications. So the first step in treating it is to come to grips with what is actually occurring. Identify it for what it is.

Next look for alternatives. Could there be an alternative reason for their pessimistic view? Is there secondary gain in their noncompliance? For example if a patient says he just can't seem to shake his back problem, could there be an ulterior motive for that? Perhaps he keeps getting narcotics because of it. Or he could be scared or in denial. A lot of patients are. Every healthcare provider knows patients who refuse to accept the truth about their health. Look for all the possible motives, causes, and explanations for their perceived pessimism, and try to understand them.

The third step is to change the perspective. If you don't know why a patient is feeling cynical, ask them. If you can get them to expand—if you can break down that shell around what you are viewing as pessimism—you will often find treasure inside. Say things like, "In order for me to help you, I need to know why you feel this way today. Please tell me. Really? That's interesting. Tell me more." Their answer may not necessarily be correct or logical, but at least you know where they're coming from.

It's hard to hold on to a perception when the foundational cause for that perception has changed. It's hard for a patient to cling to their pessimism when the real reason is exposed and discredited. For example I've had patients tell me they can't afford to join a health club, so I offered to pay their entrance fees if they would join me at the gym the next morning at 5:00. I told them if they did it for three days in a row, I would pay for the entire month. I have yet to have anybody take me up on it. They have reasons for why they don't want to exercise, for why they don't want to participate. Busy schedules top the list. I have busy days too. However, I make time to wake up at 5:00 a.m. and go to the gym. I make the time to prepare a lean turkey sandwich for my brown-bag lunch instead of stopping at the fast food place for a greasy burger. Everybody's got their reasons. You just have to get them into a fresh perspective.

Then it's time for step number four: get them to swallow a gratitude pill. Remind them to be grateful for what they *do* have. Some people are sad cases. Some people have been dealt a bad hand of cards in life, and it sucks for them. Everybody has something to overcome. But if they managed to wake up alive this morning, they have something to be thankful for. Offer them that positive thought. At least throw something constructive out there; offer some little prescription for the patient's pessimism.

Now I want to flip-flop this because I think there is an even bigger ailment in the world today, and it is pessimism among healthcare providers. I know our profession is a pressure cooker. Burnout occurs for good reason, and it's largely due to cynicism and pessimism. You see it all the time. You read about it. You've watched it happen to your colleagues (and maybe even yourself) over the years. We're all susceptible to it. If you're feeling pessimistic right now, this book is here to treat you. Have faith; know that when the symptoms are caught early enough, they can be neutralized by the antibodies for pessimism: confidence, optimism, and trust. So let's start over with you on the examining table.

Step number one: Confront reality. Recognize it. Are you being realistic and pragmatic? Or are you, in the words of my ten-year-old daughter, just being a poop head? Doctors are notorious for always trying to be realistic, but there's a fine line between pragmatism and pessimism. Look well before you leap across that line.

The second step is to ask yourself what the real problem is. If you think you hate being in the clinic, what is at the heart of that? Is it the patients you don't want to see? Are you bored? Are you feeling bad medically? If so is it because you stopped exercising? Do you have troubles at home that are carrying over and causing frustration during the day? What is the root issue? You must address whatever it is before you can be happy and fulfilled again.

Third: perspective, perspective, perspective. You're about to walk into the exam room to see a patient you've counseled for years to quit smoking, yet she has refused to comply. You have had it up to *here* with her. You're thinking, *What's the point of this?*

Nobody ever listens to me. Why do I waste my breath? Stop. Is that patient's smoking truly the reason your blood is boiling right now? Is that really a sufficient reason for you to be miserable and to be rude to your staff? Is that a good enough reason to leave in a huff and take an extra half hour at lunch, and set your entire clinic behind because you just don't want to go back? It's not.

When that happens step back and know that what you are doing is noble. You are there to provide care. Sometimes all you can do is all you can do. Continue to recommend the right thing to your smokestack patient and then move on with your life.

Which leads me to step number four: be grateful. A shot of gratitude can get you over just about any mountain — even the imaginary ones. I have a colleague who is a very shrewd investor and makes more than a million dollars a year. By anyone's standards he is quite well off. Still, he complains nonstop and stews in his own misery about the inevitable healthcare changes that are taking place and how he is certain they are going to ruin his business. Every morning when I come into the surgery center, there he is griping about the new legislation and getting so angry I can see the veins bulging in his neck. I am always tempted to say, "Oh my goodness, you poor thing! Are you going to be able to pull through? Are your kids eating bread and water now? God forbid you may have to sell one of your many office buildings and go live under a bridge!"

It's just plain silly.

Embrace change as best you can. It's what we must do as doctors. Our reward is in the ability to do what we do, not in the ability to collect on it. Whenever thoughts of impending doom (real or imagined) hit you, step back and be grateful for whatever is right in front of you. It's the only sure way to stay in this moment, and this moment is all we've got. It's the only thing we can control. So if you got out of bed this morning and you can see, hear, walk, and take a deep breath, then stop being pessimistic and cynical because many folks — including many of the ones you will be privileged to help today — cannot.

ACTION POINTS

1. *Pessimism is a disease state and it makes people sick. Recognize it. Is it realism or pessimism?*

2. *Seek out the reason for pessimism (in your patient or yourself) and put it into the perspective of that for which you deserve to be grateful.*

3. *If you don't like a situation, take action to change it. If you have no control over the situation, then you may as well cheer up and make your patient (and yourself) feel better.*

4. *In the words of a ten-year-old girl, "Life's too short to be a poop head."*

The Lake Wobegon Effect

Conceit is bragging about yourself. Confidence means
you believe you can get the job done.

— JOHNNY UNITAS

Lake Wobegon, Minnesota, is the fictional hometown of humorist Garrison Keillor, who, in his weekly radio show, *A Prairie Home Companion*, describes Lake Wobegon as "the little town that time forgot and the decades cannot improve...where all the women are strong, all the men are good-looking, and all the children are above average." That line cracks me up every time I hear it. It's a point of view everybody can relate to. We all can name groups that consistently overrate their positive qualities. Heck, you likely belong to one. I know I do—I'm a surgeon.

In a nod to Garrison Keillor, psychologists have nicknamed this natural human tendency to overestimate our abilities the *Lake Wobegon effect*. It has also been called *illusory superiority*, the *above-average effect*, and *self-enhancement bias*. If you have ever received a friend's or relative's holiday letter filled with a glowing description of the past year's events, you've experienced the Lake Wobegon effect. In holiday letters everyone is gorgeous, gifted, successful, and popular.

"...and we were delighted (but not the least bit surprised!) that our Suzie will be dancing with the New York City ballet this summer! And son Chad's elite soccer team (he's their top scorer) will be traveling to England in March to compete in the World Junior Soccer Championship Series! College scouts are already beating down our door, most notably those from Harvard, Princeton, and Yale. Mike was named Anytown Realty's top-selling agent for the fifth year in a row. And as the recently elected chair of the Greater Anytown Community Do-Gooder Foundation, I've had a super-busy year too. Still, we managed to carve out time to ski Aspen, attend the Queen's Diamond Jubilee (had tea with Princess Kate—darling girl!), and sail the Caribbean on Anytown Realty's new yacht, the SS *Cha-Ching*...."

You get the idea. It's like when your husband swears his latest DIY home-improvement project will be completed on time and under budget. That's a self-enhancement bias if I've ever heard one.

I bring up the Lake Wobegon effect because it impacts your patients, and it is in your best interests to understand it well. Like the husband who swears he can completely retile the master bathroom in a weekend, your patients think they are much better patients than they actually are. They believe they will comply with your recommendations more than they actually will. It's good to remember that so you can hold their feet to the fire if they don't follow through. Just know that they are probably not intentionally lying to you when they swear they will walk three miles a day every day, uphill both ways, for six weeks straight until their next appointment. They honestly believe they will. That's just the Lake Wobegon effect talking.

Before you become too smug, let me remind you that as a healthcare provider, the Lake Wobegon effect also applies to you. You don't know everything. I know you think you do, but you don't. So it is OK to show your patients that you are fallible in some small measure, that you are human, and that you are trying—especially when you've come to the end of your understanding on a topic. It is perfectly acceptable to reveal that you have exhausted your options for a patient and that your tank is empty. That shows the patient that not only have you tried, but you also have run to the end with them.

Don't try to explain something you know nothing about, please. Magicians Penn and Teller have a name for that: *bullshit*. When you don't know something, admit it. It is OK to say, "That is not within my specialty. Let me look that up," or, "That's interesting. I need to do more research into that." If you aren't certain of the dose, tell the patient you're going to stop and confirm it. If you need to refer a patient to a doctor with more expertise than you possess in a particular area, do it. That will gain you far more respect than dumping a load of phony superiority all over your patient's head.

ACTION POINTS

1. *The Lake Wobegon effect is the natural human tendency to overestimate our abilities. It occurs in both patients and healthcare providers. Be mindful of it.*

2. *Bear in mind that patients will overestimate the likelihood of their compliance with recommendations. Recommend accordingly.*

3. *Avoid the Lake Wobegon effect by not trying to explain something you know nothing about. Confirm to your patients your wish to know more and then do your research or refer accordingly.*

Gossip Is Not Communication

*Fire and swords are slow engines of destruction
compared to the tongue of a Gossip.*

— RICHARD STEELE

If there is one positive that has come out of the Health Insurance Portability and Accountability Act (HIPAA), perhaps it is that gossip has gone down dramatically during doctor-patient interactions. There is nothing communicative about gossiping in a medical setting. Not only are you subjecting yourself and your patient to the phenomenon of spontaneous trait transference (the boomerang effect, as we discussed in a previous chapter), but you are also making everybody within earshot feel bad.

Your patients come to you to feel better. So if you hear or read something embarrassing about a patient, keep it to yourself.

"Bob, I read about your DUI arrest in the paper last week," you say, "and I want to say I'm sorry about that, and I'm here to help you."

Oh no. No, no, no. You are not helping Bob, believe me. Don't bring it up, even if you are sincerely hoping to reassure him. The only thing Bob is going to hear is the negative. The only thing he's going to feel is shame. He is there for medical care. You're there to make him feel better whether it's through your communication skills, your medical knowledge, or your surgical expertise. Don't embarrass your patient that way.

Sometimes patients will bring up divisive local or national issues, political situations, or religious topics. Don't get dragged into any of it. If they mention the recent newspaper article about a prominent person with financial troubles or the local celebrity who's having an affair, act as if you haven't heard about it. Say, "I don't know about that" and steer the conversation back to patient care. Remember the three monkeys—hear no evil, see no evil, speak no evil? Be the monkeys. It doesn't matter who is messing around with whom or who is facing impending business doom. That's gossip; it's not medicine.

The same holds true—and I can't stress this enough—for demeaning jokes and off-color humor. Hate it! There are always going to be patients who think what they're saying is funny when it's not. If it is demeaning to or judgmental of another person based on their skin color, sexuality, religion, nationality, or disability then it is no joke. There is nothing funny about prejudice. Don't participate. Eliminate the proverbial "courtesy chuckle" from your repertoire when you hear intolerant speech. There is nothing courteous about laughing alongside a bigot.

To move on from an uncomfortable situation, you can try to save your patients from themselves. Let's say a patient starts telling a joke. As soon as it becomes apparent to you that the joke is headed in a prejudicial direction, say, "Hey, I have to stop you right there," or, "I feel like I have to interrupt here," or, "I'll take a pass on hearing things like that today," or, "No, no. Thank you for stopping. Let's move on." It's OK to do that. Don't worry about hurting their feelings or embarrassing them. If they choose to perpetuate bigotry, they deserve to be embarrassed. That's my personal opinion. Do that patient a favor and stop him from saying something you know to be wrong. If a patient started to light up a cigarette in your clinic room, would you stop her? Of course you would. You know it's wrong. You know smoking is not appropriate in a medical setting. In the same way you would stop her from spewing cigarette smoke throughout your office environment, you should feel free to stop her from spewing ugly words.

Be warm. Be friendly. But be firm. Do not participate in gossip or prejudice.

ACTION POINTS

1. *Remember your obligation to the Health Information Portability and Accountability Act and do not participate in gossip.*

2. *Steer the conversation toward positive circumstances and patient care. Saying bad things about someone else is never helpful.*

3. *There is nothing funny about prejudice. If what the patient is saying is demeaning to or judgmental of another person based on race, sexuality, religion, nationality, or disability, do not participate, and redirect immediately.*

Because. Now. Imagine.

Thaw, with her gentle persuasion, is more powerful than Thor with his hammer. The one melts; the other breaks into pieces.

— Henry David Thoreau

Since so much of being a healthcare provider is about convincing patients to do things they don't want to do, it is important to choose your words carefully and frame your recommendations properly. Saying power words like *because, now,* and *imagine* makes your sentences more potent and authoritative, but in a kinder, gentler, less obtrusive way. These words magically intensify your influence with no arm twisting required. *Because, now,* and *imagine* will definitely help you become more persuasive with your patients. Let's break it down.

Using the word *because* is a great technique when you request something from your patients because people long to understand reasons. We always want to know why. Reasons and explanations are the conscious mind's way of making sense of the world. When a child asks his mother if he can have a cookie and Mom says "no," what does the child almost always say in response?

"Why not?"

Mom's reply: "Because I said so."

Once Mom says that, the conversation is over. Granted, "I said so" isn't much of a reason, but studies show that simply using the word *because* legitimizes whatever comes after it—even if it is as lame as "I said so." In the late 1970s, Harvard psychologist Ellen Langer et al. conducted fascinating research[23] showing that when we ask someone to do us a favor, we get more compliance when we provide a reason for our request even if that reason is utter nonsense. In the study an actor asked if she could cut in front of another person to use a busy office copy machine. The actor was instructed to make the request using one of three prepared statements. The first statement was, "Excuse me. May I use the copy machine?" The compliance rate for that statement was around 60 percent. But when the actor used the second statement, "Excuse me. May I use the copy machine because I'm in a rush?" the compliance rate jumped to nearly 95 percent.

It's easy to assume that the compliance rate went sky high in the second example because the actor expressed a legitimate reason (urgency) for needing the machine, but Langer and her colleagues wanted to test that theory to be certain. So they had the actor butt into line again, but this time her prepared statement was, "Excuse me, may I use the copy machine because I have to make copies?"

That's a pretty ridiculous excuse, right? *Everybody* has to make copies—that's why they were all standing in line at the copy machine. But guess what? Even with that nonsensical, illogical excuse for wanting to cut into the line, the compliance rate remained at almost 95 percent.

The word *because* empowers even the silliest justifications for whatever follows, so use it in conversation with your patients whenever you can:

"I'd like you to take this blood pressure medication because...."

---

23 Ellen Langer, Arthur Blank, and Benzion Chanowitz, "The Mindlessness of Ostensibly Thoughtful Action: The Role of 'Placebic' Information in Interpersonal Interaction," *Journal of Personality and Social Psychology* 36, 6 (1978): 635–42.

"I recommend exercising three or four times a week because...."

You can even say, "Take this antibiotic until it's gone because I want you to take it until it's gone." You and I both know that doesn't make any sense. Still, Langer's research shows that your compliance rate will be more than 94 percent if you do. What if 94 percent of all of our recommendations in the medical field were followed? How fantastic would that be? I don't think we approach even fifty percent compliance when it comes to patients following our recommendations for exercise, quitting smoking, diet, and things like that. If you could nearly double your compliance rate by simply offering one well-placed word, why wouldn't you?

Now for the word *now*. This one is quite similar to *because*. *Now* is a courteous but authoritative motivator for most folks, and again the root of it goes way back to our childhoods.

"It's time to go to bed, Johnny."

"But Mom! I don't want to."

"Son, you have to go to bed."

"Mom, but—"

"Now!"

Remember when your mom said that? That was the end of the conversation. Case closed. *Now* elevates the importance of the message:

"Mrs. Smith, I'd like you to take this blood pressure medicine *now because* you are at risk for heart attack."

"Bob, I want you to begin eating more green leafy vegetables *now because* it will make you stronger."

"Mr. Smith, I want you to step up your physical therapy *now because* your shoulder needs more flexibility."

Then we come to the word *imagine*. This is a great power word because there is usually no resistance associated with it. Asking a patient to imagine something positive plants a seed in their mind—a seed that just might sprout into something beautiful someday. For example if you say, "Mrs. Smith, I want you to go for a walk five times a week," there might be some fairly strong hostility toward that idea. Mrs. Smith will immediately think of all the reasons why she can't walk that often: her back hurts, she doesn't have the time, or she simply doesn't want to.

But if you ask her to *imagine* herself enjoying a walk, she will probably have no opposition. When she gets home from her appointment, she may even start daydreaming about the act of walking. Those daydreams may eventually inspire her to go buy some cool new walking shoes, download some motivational music onto her mobile device, and actually hit the road.

So say things to your patients like:

"Bob, imagine if you could run up the stairs without effort."

"Imagine if your knee didn't hurt anymore."

"Imagine if you could raise your arm above your head without shoulder pain."

One of the most successful car advertising slogans in history was "imagine yourself in a Mercury now." Inspire your patients to imagine themselves with better health and they might actually take steps to make it happen.

Hey, if worked for Mercury, it can work for you.

ACTION POINTS

1. *Inserting the word* because *after your recommendation and before the reason (any reason) will greatly increase compliance with your recommendation.*

2. *Use the word* now *when you want your patients to take prompt action on a recommendation. It is a known motivator and adds a sense of urgency.*

3. *Ask your patient to* imagine *a positive result of your recommendations. Doing so plants a positive image in the patient's mind.*

Embedded Commands and Metaphors

*Metaphors have a way of holding the most truth
in the least space.*

— ORSON SCOTT CARD

Nobody likes being called a manipulator, and nobody likes to be manipulated. But theoretically all verbal communication is manipulation to some degree. For us healthcare professionals, our number one task is to manipulate our patients into being healthy. We're trying to sell people on health and wellness — on being better. Embedded commands and metaphors can help us make that sale.

An embedded command is a covert suggestion entrenched within a larger communication. You can use embedded commands to improve your relationship with a patient and to improve their quality of life. You want to present these commands in a subtle way. There are five ways to do that.

First, *know what you want to say.* Usually you have a plan with every patient. You know why they are there — for a check-up, a follow-up, surgery, those types of things. Understand the context of the visit and know exactly what it is you want the patient to do.

Number two is *the candy wrapper*. To help your patients improve and to help you improve, you must deliver your suggestion in a positive way by wrapping it inside a comment that promotes a good feeling. Study the previous sentence, because that's a real-world example of what I'm talking about. I stated, "To help your patients improve…to help you improve…positive…a good feeling." That's the candy wrapper.

Third, *choose your marker*. A marker can be a change in your speaking tempo. It can be pausing right before an important word. It can be a tone change — usually a downward inflection. But most often it's using nonverbal markers like hand movements, an eyebrow raise, a nod of the head, leaning in toward the patient, tapping your fingers together when you say certain commands, or the upper-arm touch we covered in a previous chapter. Markers help register your commands with the patient.

Fourth, *practice*. As healthcare providers we practice everything we do. We practice surgery. We practice reading EKGs when we're in medical school. We practice running other tests and understanding them. Practice communicating with patients and using embedded commands.

And fifth, *take action*. It doesn't work if you don't do it. Try it.

Let me give you an example involving getting a patient to do physical therapy after knee surgery. First I have to understand exactly what I want the patient to do: I want to get him to do his physical therapy after surgery as prescribed. And I know exactly what I want to communicate: I want to tell him what the positive outcomes of doing physical therapy after knee surgery will be. I want to tell him that his doctor will benefit and he will benefit if he does the therapy.

Number two, the candy wrapper: "Imagine, John, how it would feel when you can bend that knee without pain. Imagine a time when you will easily run up a set of stairs. Imagine you can play outside with your grandchildren and how fantastic that would be." That's the candy wrapper of *you can* and *you will* benefit from doing the physical therapy.

Third, pick a marker. Perhaps there will be a subtle clap of the hands or a gentle tap of the fingers together with your embedded commands.

Now we have to practice, which is the fourth step. In the following sentence, I've accentuated the embedded commands with asterisks and italicized print:

"Mr. Smith, your knee will *feel fantastic* after we complete this plan. When *you do your exercises *every day*, your knee gets *stronger* and *stronger*. Physical therapy will *improve flexibility* and get your knee feeling great. Our *success* depends on our working together. I know we can, and you will be *glad you did*."

If you tap your fingers together every time you hit an asterisk, you will embed those commands even deeper into your patient's psyche. That is neurolinguistic programming at its most basic. *Try it today* and *you will* be *amazed* by the *fantastic results *you can achieve*. (Sorry, I couldn't resist.)

Another way to improve your patient compliance rate is to use metaphors as often as you can. Patients love metaphors, and so do doctors. For example, in the specialty of pathology, metaphors are universally used to describe anomalies. *This has a cobblestone appearance, this has a mashed-potatoes appearance,* or *this has the appearance of stuck-on clay.* Everyone knows what you're talking about when you say it with a metaphor. If you say to a colleague, "We're spinning our wheels here," instantly they understand that the car is going nowhere. In their mind they can probably even see an image of a car with spinning wheels. Some people are auditory and need only to hear something to absorb it. Some people do better looking at verbiage on a page. Still others need to see pictures either real or imagined. Metaphors are especially helpful to them. Everybody is different, but it's a safe bet that most people will benefit from hearing a good metaphor.

The more you use them, the better your outcomes will be. You could simply tell Mrs. Smith that she needs to lose weight and get healthier, or you could spice up the conversation with some well-placed visual cues that really drive home your point:

"Mrs. Smith, if you're tired of feeling this way, put down the baggage of being overweight. Help yourself open the door to a life where your blood sugars are stable and your energy is sky high. This is going to be a rough road. It's going to be like walking up stairs, trying to shed this weight. Just hold on to the railing for support. That's why I'm here. I will help you climb that staircase. We'll go together."

Maybe that sounds over the top, but so what? As long as Mrs. Smith gets the message and is duly inspired to take appropriate action to save her own life, it's worth a little theatrical maneuvering on your part, don't you think?

ACTION POINTS

1. *Use embedded commands within your recommendations to increase patient compliance. (A) Know what you want to convey. (B) Wrap the point with positive words and phrases. (C) Accentuate your embedded commands with a physical marker for emphasis. (D) Practice using embedded commands. (E) The more embedded commands you practice, the more effective they become.*

2. *Use easily visualized metaphors whenever possible to illustrate your recommendations and the reasons for making them more clearly.*

Celebrate Uniqueness

Be yourself; everyone else is taken.

— Oscar Wilde

It is fun to be a doctor. You just have to find the uniqueness in each of your patients. The only way to uncover their uniqueness is to ask. Taking a patient's history is the perfect opportunity to do a little digging. You can ask a patient, "Tell me about your level of activity," or you can ask, "What do you do for fun?" You're essentially asking the same thing, but the second question is much more likely to provoke an interesting response.

I once asked a patient what he did for fun, and he replied, "I'm the mascot for our city's pro baseball team." (In the interest of confidentiality, I won't divulge the team. I will say he was a funny-looking, very young bear. But back to my point....) By asking him that question, I instantly discovered something cool about him. That led me to commend the team's latest win and to say how much I enjoyed watching them play. Voila! Instant doctor-patient rapport.

When you uncover a patient's uniqueness and celebrate it, you are doing so to your advantage and your patient's. He knows you will remember him the next time he comes in, and that makes him feel like a valued customer.

To encourage patients to disclose interesting information, ask open-ended questions. Asking, "Do you have kids?" is not going to get you nearly as far as, "Tell me about your family." Asking, "What do you do for a living?" is not going to stimulate as detailed a response as, "Tell me what you like most about your work." Frame it in a positive way and pull out some uniqueness.

When a patient tells you something unique about himself or herself, write it down. Add it to the chart list and be sure to bring it up at the next visit.

Along the same vein, look at the patient. Are they wearing anything unique? Mention it. You may not personally think it's stylish. You may not be inclined to wear something like that yourself. That's not the issue. The issue is that the patient must be proud of it or they wouldn't be wearing it. Say, "By the way, that bracelet sure is interesting," or "What cool boots!" They will be delighted that you noticed. You just moved the needle on the "my doctor is awesome" meter.

You should celebrate individuality not only in your patients but also in your office. If I asked a random group of people to envision a doctor's office, most of them would describe it as white, with a strange smell, a sliding glass window, a waiting room, and magazines. What's unique about that?

A unique office is full of smiles. It has an interesting décor or a distinctive way of greeting patients. That's all patient communication, whether it's done verbally or nonverbally. Making your patient communications unique sets you apart from the doctor down the street.

In my office we allow the front-desk personnel to dress up on Halloween. That always provokes some smiles when people walk into the office. On the day before our local college rivals play their big game, I buy a giant sandwich from the sub shop and host a tailgate lunch for my coworkers. Everybody is invited to wear their favorite college colors that day. Believe me, that gets people talking. It doesn't matter which team everyone's rooting for. It opens people up and distinguishes our office from the rest of the pack.

Who's the most creative person in your office? Who's quirky? Who's funny? Who's unique? Ask them for ideas for making your office a more interesting place. Just because you're the doctor, nurse practitioner, or PA doesn't mean you know everything. Reach out. Look for new ways to make your office and your interactions with your staff more interesting for patients.

The more cynical among you may be thinking, *Patients aren't there to enjoy. It's not supposed to be fun to go to the doctor.* Well, why not? What do you mean? It's not fun to feel better? It's not fun to smile? Fun and smiling are important. For far too long, we healthcare providers have been caught up in the dogma that ours is a professional environment and it needs to remain that way. But I believe we need to move on from that and find the middle ground between the extremes of stuffy formality and wild abandon.

And that leads me to Thorndike's law. American psychologist Edward Thorndike once wrote:

> *Responses that produce a satisfying or pleasant state of affairs in a particular situation are more likely to occur again in a similar situation. Conversely, responses that produce a discomforting, annoying or unpleasant effect are less likely to occur in that same situation again.*[24]

That is what's called *Thorndike's law of effect.* In a nutshell it means that pleasant experiences are more likely to be repeated; unpleasant ones are not. So if you want a patient never to return to your office, never to honor your recommendations, or never to refer another patient to you then by all means make them uncomfortable by staring at your computer while you talk to them. Annoy them by standing behind their wheelchair so they have to strain their neck to look at you. Be perceived as generally unpleasant by never smiling or thanking them for coming in. And for heaven's sake, never celebrate their uniqueness or allow any uniqueness whatsoever to creep into your office.

---

24 Peter Gray, *Psychology*, Sixth Edition (Worth Publishers, 2011), 109.

The bottom line is if you want satisfying outcomes and fewer lawsuits then satisfy your patients' hunger for a caring, outgoing, unique healthcare provider—one who smiles, says "thank you," celebrates their individuality, and makes their visits pleasant. That's not just my opinion. It's the law. Thorndike's law of effect, that is.

ACTION POINTS

1. *Ask open-ended questions to discover something unique about your patient. Celebrating a patient's uniqueness is rapport building at its finest.*

2. *Make your work environment distinctive and interesting. A unique office is full of smiles, interesting décor, and a fresh way of greeting patients.*

3. *Thorndike's law of effect says that pleasant experiences are more likely to be repeated; unpleasant ones are not. If you want patients to return, honor your recommendations, and provide referrals, then make their visits with you pleasant experiences.*

Medical Office Feng Shui

Peace is always beautiful.

— WALT WHITMAN

In 2009 the European Agency for Safety and Health at Work estimated that stress causes up to 50 percent of the absenteeism in the workplace.[25] In 2004 the American Institute of Stress stated that work-related stress and accidents accounted for up to 75 percent of absenteeism and led to nearly $300 billion in lost productivity and employee turnover.[26]

As physicians and healthcare providers, we already know that stress causes illness and loss of productivity. That's just common sense. And if we know that stress causes harm, we're shooting ourselves in the feet if we don't eliminate the environmental causes of stress in our own offices. Failing to do so goes against

25 Malgorzata Milczarek, Elke Schneider, Eusebio Rial González, "European Risk Observatory Report: OSH in Figures: Stress at Work—Facts and Figures," European Agency for Safety and Health at Work, accessed March 23, 2013, https://osha.europa.eu/en/publications/reports/TE-81-08-478-EN-C_OSH_in_figures_stress_at_work.

26 The American Institute of Stress, "Workplace Stress," accessed March 23, 2013, www.stress.org/workplace-stress.

every tenet of medical care because we're supposed to be helping people prevent and cure illnesses, not causing them.

Recognize that you are not the only one communicating with your patients and staff every day. Your building and rooms are communicating something as well. What is your office environment saying to your staff when they walk in? Is it a pleasant place to work or is it irritating and discordant, like fingernails on a chalkboard? What is your office environment saying to your patients when they walk in? Is it, "Good morning! Welcome! We're glad you're here!" Or, "We're so unorganized around here! Go have a seat over there and we'll be with you in an hour...if you're lucky."

Your office and its appearance communicate to your patients. Your office is, in essence, an extension of the care you are offering them.

The difference between a good restaurant and a great restaurant is in the details, and the same holds true for a medical office. Start addressing those details by putting yourself in your patients' and staff's shoes. The next time you go to your physician's office or to see your physician's assistant or nurse practitioner, walk in with a different set of eyes. Sit down with the environment in mind. It's not about you this time; it's about the space you're in. What cues are you picking up? Specifically which features of the space relax you? What annoys you? Take notes.

Then go into your own office environment and conduct the same analysis. Sit down in the reception area and look around. Observe the environment at different times during the day if you can. If you can't, have someone unknown to the staff — perhaps a friend, or a coworker of your spouse — do the same thing and report back about what they felt was good and not so good about the reception area.

By the way, what do you call that space? You can call it either a "waiting room" or a "relaxation area." The former screams that patients are going to have to wait in this office, while the latter suggests they are going to relax. I encourage changing the name of that room. Get everyone in your office to refer to it as the "relaxation area." Toss out the old sign that says "waiting room" and replace it with warm, inviting smiles.

Look at the desks. Look at the walls. Look at the ceilings. Are there stains on the tiles? Walk down the hallways. Are there stains on the carpet? Is it worn? Does the décor match? Does it flow? Is the lighting harsh? What about sound—can you hear someone talking about their elderly mother's illness from another room?

What follows is a list of basic environmental principles, grounded in Chinese feng shui, that can be incorporated into a medical office. I'm not saying that every one of these suggestions will be appropriate for your office, but they are things that have been shown to be helpful in promoting relaxation and well-being in a variety of settings. However, before we get started, one quick word about office décor: no matter what you do, make sure it's tasteful. Make sure it's not over the top. Nothing says "I am taking way too much money from my patients" like expensive, Victorian statues in the corners and gold-inlaid travertine tile floors. Strive for beautiful, but stop well shy of extravagant.

With that out of the way, let's begin with color. Many medical settings are all white or all gray, which is stress-inducing. White and gray rooms feel stark, indifferent, and cold. There is no reason to perpetuate this unbearable whiteness of being in our offices. It doesn't change a room's sterility to paint it something other than white or gray. Instead choose from a soothing color palette that echoes the earth, water, and wood elements in feng shui. Earth colors—light yellow, olive green, beige, and sand—promote feelings of nourishment and stability. Watery colors in soothing shades of blue stimulate feelings of tranquility and purity. Wood colors, such as soft browns and greens, foster an aura of vitality, wellness, and growth. You can incorporate brighter colors as accents, but keep the overall background palette calm. Paint is cheap and can be changed easily, so experiment and have fun with it.

Introduce a few live plants into the space. Every room benefits from plants. They bring fresh energy and help purify the air. Just make sure they are well kept. Nothing says "despair to all who enter here" like a sick plant withering away in the corner. How can you expect your patients to believe that you can take care of them properly when you can't even keep a plant alive? If you have to, hire an expert to maintain your little indoor container garden, so be it. Also, avoid sharp plants. Don't put a cactus in the middle of the room. They don't make people think comfortable thoughts. Bring in flowing, lush plants that are fun to look at. Don't overdo it, though. You don't want your relaxation area to look like a jungle. Less is more.

Introduce a water element. Studies show that flowing water is stress-relieving. People relax when they hear it. That's why so many folks have those relaxation machines that play sounds of rain and ocean waves. Many dentists' offices have fish tanks. Watching fish swim is relaxing. Hearing the sound of gurgling water is soothing. Even if a fish tank won't work in your office, you can still set up some type of flowing-water feature such as a fountain on a wall, floor, or tabletop. Again, put someone in charge of keeping it crystal clean. Fountains can get nasty if neglected. Don't ask me how I know this.

Arrange the furniture in a way that makes people feel comfortable. No one should have to sit with their back to a doorway, particularly a main entrance. When a person's back is to the entrance of the room, they feel vulnerable. They feel the constant need to turn around to maintain their own internal security. Exam tables are no exception. If you don't believe me, sit in an exam room on a table with your back to the door and see how it feels to wonder who just came in. Be sure to be naked except for a crinkly paper gown when you conduct this experiment. It is not a pleasant feeling. So turn those tables toward the door. If you don't want to have the end of the table facing the door—in a gynecology office, for example—then put up a curtain you can draw during exams. Give the patient the security of knowing that they can see the entrance and exit at all times.

In the relaxation room (formerly known as the waiting room), arrange the sofas and chairs in such a way that nobody has to sit with their back to a pass-through area. It is uncomfortable to sit in a chair when other people are walking around behind you. You can't tell what's going on back there without turning around, and you don't want to turn around all the time because it makes you look paranoid. That is not a relaxing way to spend five minutes, let alone an hour or more. Help your patients. Don't put them through that discomfort.

Lighting is an important part of every room, and thankfully it is a very simple thing to adjust. Fluorescent lighting is harsh, so replace it. The more natural, full-spectrum light you can bring in — like sunlight, for instance — the better. If you're in a high-rise and can't get much sunlight in the room, then introduce full-spectrum light using table and floor lamps, up-lights around plants, gallery lights over artwork, track lighting, and/or hanging lamps.

Studies show that when people see circles or rounded edges, they are more at ease in comparison to when they see sharp corners. It is easier for the brain to process rounded shapes. Therefore the tables and containers in your office should be round or oval.

Ditch the clutter. Messy stacks of paperwork and dusty knick-knacks on desks and tables are indications of sloppiness. Masses of tangled cables, wires, cords, plugs, power strips, and other industrial-looking items suggest turmoil. Sloppiness and turmoil are not what you want to convey in a medical setting. By taking steps to clear the clutter in areas that are visible to your patients, you are also taking steps to clear their minds and make them feel more at ease.

What's more inviting: a cookie jar with two cookies and crumbs in the bottom or a full-to-overflowing cookie jar? An empty container conveys exactly that — emptiness, desolation, and barrenness. You, however, want to convey a sense of richness and abundance in your office. So if you have any visible containers in your clinic room, in the relaxation area, or on the reception desk, keep them full. If it's a container filled with smooth river stones, fill it all the way to the top. If it's a bowl of mints on the reception desk, keep it stocked at all times.

I know that fans are not an option in certain medical offices, particularly in settings in which sterility is a major issue. In other types of settings, a fan may be a good addition to a room or suite of offices. I'm not talking about a floor fan that blows air directly at people. I'm referring to circulating fans that simply keep air moving around the room.

People prefer fresh air over stale air. Ask anyone what a medical office smells like and they'll give you an answer we all know: medical offices smell like disinfectant. Maybe it's a good thing that our offices smell clean, but sometimes it can be overwhelmingly medicinal. If you have the option, consider using aromatherapy in your office. The scents of lavender and chamomile are believed to stimulate relaxation. Studies show that the scent of sandalwood puts people at ease and even makes them more likely to buy things. If you don't believe me, go into any Bath & Body Works, Victoria's Secret, or Abercrombie & Fitch and sniff the air. There is a compelling (financial) reason why they don't smell like industrial cleaners.

Whether or not to have a television in the relaxation area is a big question mark. I wish you wouldn't. But if you are determined to have one, tune it to something that is pleasant to watch, and keep the volume low. If your practice caters to adults, HGTV (Home and Garden Television) is probably safe. For pediatrics a G-rated movie on DVD (no commercials!) is your best bet. The goal is to be innocuous — to make sure that whatever you're showing will not irritate anyone. Remember, they're a captive audience. Treat them kindly.

The same holds true for the magazines we commonly find in medical offices. You have a choice in the kinds of publications you offer, so be thoughtful when making that choice. Your patients want to have something to look at, but they don't want to read about Kim Jong-un and the next North Korean rocket. The magazine cover shot of the latest war refugees is not a calming image. You can choose to have *People* magazine and Jersey Shore gossip or you can choose to have periodicals about wellness, stress relief, and feeling better. It's entirely up to you. Just remember that your relaxation area gives you a superb opportunity to communicate with your patients by setting out material that adds value to their day.

I know of one surgery center that has little boxes of Trivial Pursuit cards on the tables in the waiting area. Those are a blast for people to look at. The patients learn something, and the cards are great conversation starters. I've seen strangers connect with one another over those cards, making their waiting time seemingly fly by. It's nice to offer your patients an opportunity like that.

Music is another way to put people at ease. But be careful: picking the right music can be quite a dilemma. Everybody has different tastes. Some people like classical music, others like soft rock, still others relax by listening to opera. I believe you can't go wrong with purely instrumental spa music. You can go on iTunes and find thousands of songs to choose from and download. You can even find spa music with subliminal messages of health, relaxation, and well-being embedded in them. That's certainly an easy thing to offer within your clinic. I think music beats TV hands down when it comes to promoting calm and peace in your office.

One caveat, though: be conscious of the fact that your employees have to sit and listen to that music all day every day. Be sure to let them know that they can change a particular track whenever it starts to get old. It's easy to say, "Get over it. We're here for the patients." I know; I've hammered home the message throughout this book that the patients come first. However, communicating to your employees that they matter too is a reasonable (and decent) thing to do. Give them the power to switch out the music because if you have a frustrated employee, they're probably going to frustrate your patients.

Next, consider the technical and legal considerations of HIPAA. If you're in the medical field, you know that anything with the patient's name on it should not be visible to anyone outside the practice. I can't tell you how many times I've been to a medical office where I walked up to the front desk to check in and saw a stack of patient charts sitting right there in front of me. I could easily have read the names on the files. On more than one occasion, I've seen the list of the patients set to come in that day. At the checkout desk I've also read a computer screen situated in such a way that I could see information about the last patient — including how they didn't pay their bill. Eliminate from plain sight anything with patient information on it.

Finally, give your patients something to hold on to when they're afraid or hurting. Children and adults alike feel better when they hold a stuffed animal, a fuzzy pillow, or a soft, cushy blanket. It puts them at ease immediately. In my office we have a number of little stuffed dogs and teddy bears that my patients can hold before, during, and after their procedures. Time and again patients say they're comforted by holding them. Kids of all ages should be given that option. I can tell you for a fact that the stuffed animals in our office have helped a lot more adults than kids.

ACTION POINTS

1. *You are not the only one communicating with your patients and staff every day. Your office and its appearance communicate to your patients as well. Your office is an extension of the care you offer to your patients.*

2. *Have someone you trust tell you the truth — have them "mystery shop" your office, in essence, and report back to you what your office environment is saying. Is it odd smelling, harsh, and noisy? Or is it relaxing, soothing, and conveying health and wellness?*

3. *Consider earth tones, live plants, and water elements to put patients at ease while in your office.*

4. *Evaluate the sounds (or lack thereof) in your office and consider instrumental, relaxation-based music or background-sound-generating devices to help put patients at ease.*

5. *Any item in your office that contains a patient's name should not be visible to other patients. Eliminate sign-in sheets and multiuse forms that disclose patients' names. Be mindful of files and computer screens that may be visible to other patients.*

Traction Control

For fast acting relief, try slowing down.

— LILY TOMLIN

Imagine you're walking up a steep hill. The gravel gives way beneath your feet, and you start to slip. What do you do? You certainly don't start sprinting and scurrying faster and faster. No, you slow down and look for something to grab on to in order to steady yourself. You stop and try to get some traction.

And that's exactly what you need to do sometimes when you're communicating with your patients. When we're trying hard to get through to someone to help them get better and to improve their compliance, sometimes we push harder and faster. That affects our body language and eye contact in ways that can come across as aggressive. Instead we should pull back and let our words gain some traction. Author Mark Goulston put it this way:

> *Most people up shift when they want to get through to the other person. They persuade. They encourage. They argue. They push. And in the process, they create resistance. When you [slow down] you'll do exactly the opposite — you'll listen, ask, mirror, and reflect back to people what you've heard. When you do, they will feel seen,*

understood, and felt — and that unexpected down shift will draw them to you.[27]

So if a patient appears frustrated, don't bombard their already overstimulated emotions. Pause. Being silent is like taking your foot off the gas pedal when your car's tires are spinning on ice. Slow down, back up, and acknowledge the patient's frustration. Reset the conversation by giving a large and audible exhalation. I am not talking about an exasperated sigh. I'm talking about a controlled exhalation to help you relax. You can even say, "Let's stop and exhale for a moment here. Let's just breathe. I can see you're frustrated, so let's go about this in a different way."

Occasionally tears will start to flow when you convey something a patient does not want to hear. It may not necessarily be bad news, but if it is you absolutely must slow down. Allow those tears to flow. That person is crying for a reason. It means they're stressed. You can't keep pushing and pushing and stacking even more stress on top of what they already feel. That does not help. Sometimes the best therapy is just to stop and allow the silence to occur.

Then empathize with the patient. You can say, "You're in pain, aren't you? I can tell." When you say that, they will nod their head and say, "Yes, I am." Now you two are in agreement, and when you're in agreement you can move forward with positive communication. Now you've regained traction and control. You can gain even more traction by showing that you are interested in why they're hurting. Ask them. Be curious, and make it obvious that you are. Showing the patient that you're curious about them removes the perception that you're in attack mode. Think about it: a curious dog and an attacking dog are two vastly different things, and it is easy to tell the difference between them. An attacking dog advances and doesn't stop for anything. A curious dog stops and tilts his head to one side. So tilt your head to the

---

27 Mark Goulston, *Just Listen: Discover the Secret to Getting Through to Absolutely Anyone* (AMACOM, 2009), 4.

side when you ask the patient why they're hurting or why they're frustrated. It will slow the conversation down in an instant.

You can even take some responsibility for what the patient is feeling. Goulston described this technique as an "empathy jolt," meaning an ounce of empathy offsets a ton of failure in a conversation. An example of an empathy jolt would be to state what the patient may be feeling and then inject a shot of empathy such as, "Bob, I can see you're frustrated and in pain. I'm sorry. Apparently I've let you down, because we are not getting the results and the improvement that I know we can."

Apologizing and saying that *we* are not getting the best results reinforces the idea that you and Bob are a team, and that the two of you are complicit. All of a sudden, Bob almost has to empathize with *you*. He may even try to reassure you by saying, "No, you haven't let me down. The truth is I haven't been eating as well as I should." Now the patient is the one saying exactly what you had hoped to convey all along. You didn't have to say it; the patient said it. You've just regained some traction thanks to the simple act of inserting an empathy jolt into the conversation.

Another way to regain control is to ask the patient what they believe. For example if Bob says he can't finish chemotherapy, respond by saying, "Do you truly believe that you can't?" Then pause and wait for his answer. That forces Bob to reflect on what he said to you. Now he's the one questioning himself about why he said he can't finish his treatment, not you. He is his own inquisitor. That's a very simple yet effective technique for getting the monkey off your back and putting the conversation back on the rails. Try it. You'll see.

Yet another great technique is to ask the patient's permission to do something by making a suggestion. For example you can say, "Mrs. Smith, I would like to suggest, with your permission, that we start this medication today because taking it will lower your blood pressure." When you infer that the patient has a choice in whatever you are suggesting, you lower their defenses. You eliminate any perception that you are in attack mode. People like to think that they have a choice.

And finally, saying "thank you" will help with your traction control. Say it to your patients and your team members as often as you can. And about your team: you can call the people who work with you whatever you want—your employees, your nurses, your techs—but in my office I call them my coworkers. They are working at the same time I am, and we're all striving together toward a common goal. I don't see the need to put myself above them on a pedestal by calling them my employees. You'll find that if you refer to the people around you as coworkers, and if you thank them for their hard work and dedication every chance you get, life will be a lot better in your clinic. I shouldn't have to put that in this book, but alas I've been around enough to know that not everyone in my profession has gotten the message yet. Thank your coworkers for their help. It doesn't hurt to smile at them either.

As for your patients, thank them for listening to you. Thank them for letting you administer their cortisone shots. Thank them for showing up. Those patients have allowed you to do your job. They have supported you in your quest to make them better. They've assisted you in your ability to bill the insurance company for their care. They have helped you regain your traction as a healthcare provider. All that deserves your heartfelt thanks, wouldn't you agree?

ACTION POINTS

1. *When we are trying to make a point or get through to someone, sometimes we push hard and become aggressive. When you notice this occurring, pull back, slow down, and allow yourself to regain traction in the conversation.*

2. *Empathize with the patient and verbally acknowledge his or her frustration.*

3. *Ask permission to make a suggestion or recommendations when the patient seems frustrated. This gives the patient a new sense of control.*

4. *Exude gratitude by thanking your patients whenever possible. Gratitude begets gratitude. Show your appreciation to your co-workers too. You may be the quarterback, but let them know you are all on the same team. They will be more likely to block for you…so to speak.*

How Old Is Your Patient?

Feelings of worth can flourish only in an atmosphere where individual differences are appreciated, mistakes are tolerated, communication is open, and rules are flexible — the kind of atmosphere that is found in a nurturing family.

— VIRGINIA SATIR

There is a big difference in the way we healthcare providers communicate with people from diverse age groups — or at least there should be if we hope to achieve good outcomes. In most cases your patient base is multigenerational, and generational perspectives vary. Simply recognizing that will help you communicate more effectively.

Cam Marston explained this concept better than anyone in his book entitled *Motivating the "What's In It For Me" Workforce: Manage Across the Generational Divide and Increase Profits*. In it Marston described the four generational groups in American society and recommended practical ways to improve your communications with each.

He called the first of these groups the Matures. Unfortunately this group, born from 1920 to 1945, is getting smaller and smaller as time marches on. The Matures were shaped by two major historical events: World War II and the Great Depression. These are people who appreciate hierarchical systems and militaristic-style organizations. Generally speaking these are the patients who will pretty much go along with whatever you recommend because to them you are an authority figure. Their mantra is, "Whatever you say. You're the doctor!"

If you ask these patients for the names of the medications they're taking, they often have no idea. They simply take the medications because you gave them the prescriptions. The Matures are extremely loyal, and they expect extreme loyalty from you in return. These patients will put up with poor communication for the sake of conformity. They have a strong work ethic, and they like to share their opinions on that topic. If you discuss your work ethic, they will appreciate it.

These are folks who expect a regimented approach to healthcare, and your communications with them should respect that. To build rapport with the Matures, you must lay out a well-ordered, step-by-step outline of their treatment plan and the outcomes you hope to achieve. If you make it crystal clear enough, they will smile, nod, and go along with it in most cases.

The second group Marston referred to is the Boomers, who were born from 1946 to 1964. This group is the largest of the four, currently numbering around eighty-four million and making up the biggest portion of our workforce. Boomers measure their work ethic by the time they have invested on the job. These are the folks who say, "I have been at this company for thirty-five years, and that's why I deserve this promotion." Due to that tenet, Boomers hold the majority of senior leadership positions across various industries, companies, and organizations.

Boomers expect to have total control over their lives at work and at home. Therefore they may become quickly frustrated if they don't have control in their medical care. Cancer and heart disease—two conditions notorious for stripping control away from patients—have major emotional effects on this age group. When the proverbial executive who is accustomed to having total control over every step in his day gets diagnosed with cancer and has to sit in someone else's office, march to someone else's schedule, and listen to someone else tell him how things are going to be...well, that is a person who is not going to be very comfortable. That is a person who may grasp desperately at some semblance of control even if it means being rude to you, the nurse, and the front-desk person. Maybe that's all he has.

You can help by acknowledging that perhaps that is the reason he feels the way he does. Cancer has ripped away every bit of influence he had in his life. If being rude to you is the only way he can get that feeling of power back for a moment, then simply acknowledge it and move on. Don't take it personally. If you say, "I can tell you feel a loss of control in this. That is certainly understandable under these circumstances," or, "Cancer doesn't play fair, does it?" then that patient will almost certainly shake his head and agree with you. When you get the patient to agree with you, you're communicating.

Boomers need to be allowed to make decisions about their medical care. Give them their options, then make your recommendations. Be sure to mention to them that you've invested a lot of years in your profession and that's why you are recommending this particular course of treatment. Then circle back and remind them that they have a choice in this. They'll appreciate that immensely.

Next is Generation X, which Marston described as being born from 1965 to 1980. This is when family dynamics changed big time in the United States. The days of Ward and June Cleaver left us forever during Generation X. These are the folks whose lives moved from the Vietnam War to the corporate greed of the 1980s. They have a tendency to be quite adept at adjusting to transition. They are much more adaptable than their Boomer parents and Mature grandparents.

These are people who have married but are in the midst of climbing the corporate ladder at the same time. Their children are growing and changing before their eyes. At times they can be cynical and distrustful of their employers and other authority figures — including doctors.

Marston called this group "the Prince Charles generation." They value efficiency, and they will be the most angry when you run behind. These are people who know they are stressed.

However, these are also people who are still kids at heart. They're not yet thinking of retirement. They're still in high gear and still transitioning between their high school days of wearing parachute pants and watching Don Johnson on *Miami Vice* to now entering a corporate management position.

To communicate effectively with Generation X, acknowledge that they're in the midst of transitioning and discuss that with them. By doing so you'll establish a line of communication that they are going to appreciate. Many people in this group are approaching menopause and andropause, for example. To them you can say, "You're watching your kids grow up and change. You're no exception, you know. Your body is changing too. We can work together to make these transitions easier and keep you healthy for years to come." Generation Xers will appreciate that level of understanding from you.

And then lastly Marston described the New Millennials, born from 1981 to the 2000s. These are people who were raised in relative comfort and prosperity in child-centric homes where it was not about discipline, it was about education. They were brought up in the ultimate world of political correctness. Allow me to give you an example (and a laugh) of what I mean. Their parents never ordered them to go take a bath. No, the lead up to bath time in a household with New Millennial children was a theatrical production of monumental proportions. Dad would start by asking his child (in his best Mr. Rogers imitation), "Sweetie? Would you like to take a bath now?" and Mom would clap her hands and squeal, "Oh! Yay! A baaaaath!" It was an Oscar-winning performance every night with the New Millennial kids as the appreciative audience.

New Millennials are technologically savvy, so your communications with them will likely be influenced by that. They prefer to schedule appointments online and be able to communicate with you by e-mail. For them time is as valuable as money. They tend to be less focused on accumulating financial wealth and working hard for it and more focused on accumulating their own time and nurturing their well-being. It's more about fulfillment and less about efficiency. They don't take rejection or criticism very well.

Sixty percent of this generation lived at home after graduating from college.

If you're communicating with people in this group, you'll need to step back and gain traction control by not criticizing or rejecting. Work with them. Offer them comfort. Highlight the intangible prosperity and personal fulfillment that your recommendations for their medical care will bring them. And do all that using technology whenever you can. New Millennials have come to expect that.

You can use these tips and descriptions of the four generational groups to help your communication with not only your patients but also your coworkers. Is your head nurse a Boomer and getting frustrated about having no control over the pending healthcare system changes? Is your medical assistant a New Millennial who doesn't really care whether or not she's being paged—she just wants to get the hell out of the office at five o'clock? You have to understand where these people are coming from if you expect to communicate with them effectively.

Also, consider matching the caregiver to the patient. Will an eighty-year-old man feel completely comfortable with a twenty-four-year-old female nurse? Knowing the way some eighty-year old men operate, he very well might. But it's highly likely that he won't. An eighty-year-old woman will probably not feel as comfortable with a twenty-four-year-old tech as she might with a sixty-one-year-old nurse. Your patients deserve to have someone they can relate to when they're in your office. It's OK to match caregivers to patients based on generational criteria. When you do you'll find that communication improves.

Obviously it's not always possible to pair patients with providers of the same age group. So if you are a sixty-year-old male and you're talking to a New Millennial, acknowledge the generational difference and convey your interest in the patient's point of view. It's okay to say, "It's been a while since I was in college. It must be really different now. Tell me, how's it going?" You've established a vein of communication. The patient will agree with you because he knows you're right: college is different now from how it was when you were there. That's the truth.

There needs to be more truth-telling in our offices. Respecting—and even capitalizing upon—generational differences will help bring that about.

ACTION POINTS

1. *The diversity of age groups makes a big difference in the way one communicates with a patient. Recognize that Matures, Boomers, Generation Xers, and New Millennials benefit from different means and techniques of communication.*

2. *Matures appreciate a regimented approach to healthcare, and your communication should reflect that. Lay out a well-ordered, step-by-step outline of their treatment plan and the outcomes you expect to achieve.*

3. *Boomers have a great deal of control in their lives and may become quickly frustrated if they don't have control in their medical care. Present options and then make recommendations. Acknowledge their discomfort and mention the years you have invested in learning how to help them.*

4. *Generation Xers are often in the midst of life transitions between children and parents of their own and climbing the career ladder—all while navigating midlife. Acknowledge that medical care is a means of managing transitions in one's health.*

5. *New Millennials are technologically savvy. Communicate accordingly. Convey that your recommendations are about fulfilling their needs and will help make their lives more efficient. Highlight the intangible prosperity your recommendations will bring. Do it with technology whenever you can.*

Rules for Discussing Religion and Politics with Patients

There are three things I have learned never to discuss with people: religion, politics, and the Great Pumpkin.

— Linus, from *It's the Great Pumpkin, Charlie Brown*

Rule #1: Do not discuss religion and politics with your patients. Ever.
Rule #2: See Rule #1.

ACTION POINTS

1. *Discussing religion and politics with patients is not recommended.*

Let the Ax Fall on Dead Trees

Some of us think holding on makes us strong,
but sometimes it is letting go.

— Hermann Hesse

When we took the Hippocratic oath, we pledged to do no harm. Part of doing no harm means that when a medical relationship becomes injurious for either you or the patient, it is your Hippocratic obligation to move away from that relationship. While it is our responsibility as healthcare professionals to provide medical care, we are under no legal obligation to provide every kind of care or to see every single person in the world. There are some things we cannot provide, and there are some people we cannot provide them to.

It is never easy to release a patient from your care or to remove a patient from your practice, but sometimes you simply have no choice. There are just some people in the world who are not good matches for other people in the world. Try as you might to connect with another person, sometimes your personalities, communication methods, and belief systems do not mesh. When the stars line up such that it is not a beneficial relationship for medical care, personal interaction, and good feelings, you need to move on. I'm going to give you some practical tips for how to do that.

But before I do, I want to stress three things. First, removing a patient from your practice is not something you can delegate to anyone else. Sorry to break it to you, but you have to do it yourself, and in most cases you must do it face to face—and document it accordingly.

Second, releasing a patient is not something you can do in the midst of an acute medical care situation without facing legal (and moral) ramifications. I shouldn't have to tell you that.

And third, while a doctor legally can dismiss a patient for any reason with no explanation, I think that should be your last option. The American College of Physician *Ethics Manual* states that we have "a moral duty to care for all patients," and in my opinion that means communicating with patients to the best of our ability at all times—even when it's difficult. Especially when it's difficult. There is no law that says you have to give a reason for dismissing a patient; however, if you want to dismiss a patient for no given reason and totally out of the blue, you should expect some fairly explosive fireworks.

That said, here are the legitimate reasons to release a patient:

- Persistent failure to keep scheduled appointments or adhere to agreed-upon treatment plans.
- Repeated failure to pay medical bills.
- Ongoing rude, disruptive, or unreasonable behavior.
- Habitual noncompliance.
- Falsifying or providing misleading medical history or other medical information.
- Sexually seductive behavior toward physician or staff.
- Any specific incidence of threat, violence, or criminal activity.

Obviously, before you reach that final decision to cut a patient loose, you really want to exhaust every effort to communicate with and get through to them. Try your best to set new goals. Try your best to meet that patient's needs. That's the basis of what we do for a living, so make every effort to do so. Cover all the bases. There are a couple of exceptions to that rule, however: whenever there is the threat of violence or a blatant sexual advance, you must stop the situation immediately and release the patient on the spot. Document it well and move on.

In all other cases, make sure the patient has access to other providers before you send them on their way. You can help by giving them a list of providers within their plan or a list of providers affiliated with the local medical society. You can even offer to set up their first appointment for them. Document that you gave them the list and offered to help. You can document it on paper, but you can also orally document what you did by bringing a third party into the visit with you. Perhaps a nurse or medical assistant can sit in and listen to what you're saying, especially if the patient has another person in the room with them. You must even the playing field to avoid the proverbial "he said, she said" spectacle that so often characterizes these types of discussions.

No matter what happens, remain calm. This is not a happy thing you're doing. It is not something to be taken lightly. It is a serious situation. Do it professionally. You can say something like, "It is my obligation to find you the best care possible, and it doesn't seem that I am providing that for you. You have other options, and I think that pursuing them will be in your best interest."

That will usually disarm the patient at least somewhat. However, you don't usually say things like this to patients who are rational and whom you love to see — people who are happy and a joy for everyone in the office to deal with. You usually have to say it to people who are the opposite of all those things. Therefore, expect the encounter to be unpleasant. Expect it to be a noisy, disruptive clash that could be upsetting for your coworkers and other patients who are within earshot. It is best to schedule these particular appointments at the end of the day, or perhaps make them the last appointments before the office closes for lunch. (I know, I know. "The office closes for lunch?" Yeah, right.)

Immediately after the dust has settled, send a letter to the patient reiterating what was discussed in your face-to-face meeting and offer to provide emergency care for a reasonable time while they seek out another physician. Typically that's about thirty days. You can even enclose a copy of the original list of physicians you gave them at the meeting. Then wish them good luck in their future endeavors, because they are probably going to need it.

ACTION POINTS

1. *Always make your best effort, but sometimes you simply must proactively release a patient from your care.*

   a. *Do it yourself, and in a face-to-face meeting with the patient. Document it accordingly.*

   b. *Do not release a patient in the midst of an acute or urgent medical care situation.*

   c. *Make sure the patient has access to other medical providers, and provide a list of these for the patient.*

   d. *Follow up with a letter reiterating what was discussed in your face-to-face meeting and enclose a copy of the original provider list.*

2. *Document, document, document.*

Communicating Bad News

Bad news isn't wine. It doesn't improve with age.

— COLIN POWELL

As much as we would like everybody around us to be cheerful and carefree, people don't go to the doctor because they're happy and healthy. They go to the doctor because they're hurting and troubled. Sometimes we have great outcomes and everyone goes home happy and feeling better. But unfortunately some health-care situations go from bad to worse. Complications can and do occur. The ramifications of those complications are often terrible, requiring us to deliver unpleasant news to people who were already strained to the breaking point to begin with.

Communicating bad news is a major challenge for most healthcare providers. Even some of the most seasoned doctors have difficulty with it, with the possible exception of oncologists and cancer surgeons. They are well-versed (some better than others) in the art of delivering bad news because they have to do it every day. But the rest of us are neither trained nor accustomed to giving a patient a bad report. That lack of training and experience can lead to uncomfortable situations for everyone involved. In order to help our patients and their families, it is vitally important that we learn how to work through those difficult times. It is also critical to your own well-being, mindset, and malpractice provider that you become proficient at being the bearer of bad news.

The first rule for delivering bad news is *tell the truth*. A friend of mine named Dan Sullivan founded a fantastic entrepreneur-coaching program many years ago called Strategic Coach®. I highly recommend Dan's program for anyone wanting to become a better team player, businessperson, and leader. In a seminar I once heard Dan say something that really resonated with me. He said, "All progress begins by telling the truth." I firmly believe that. In the medical environment, deception or half truths are not deception or half truths. They are lies, and lies have no role to play in medical care. Communication is an art, but medicine is a science backed up by facts. There is no such thing as a half-baked fact. You are never wrong when you are telling the truth. Unfortunately sometimes it will hurt very much to be honest. But it will always be the right thing to do.

Reveal it, don't conceal it. Don't try to hide the truth, not even for a moment. You are not protecting anyone by doing that. Avoiding a difficult conversation may make you feel better but only momentarily. If the patient and/or family find out from the nurse that something bad happened fifteen minutes ago but you haven't discussed it with them yet, it will hurt them and crush your reputation. Don't conceal the truth, not even for a short time.

Address bad news in a timely manner because you will inevitably be asked, "How long have you known this?" Do you really want to explain to the patient that you have had their lab results for three days but you've been too nervous to call? Hint: no, you don't. You can expect fireworks to occur when you say something like that. You will be judged accordingly. There is no good time to convey bad news, of course, but sooner is always better than later.

When it's time to deliver the bad news, *establish rapport* with the patient or family using some of the tips we've already covered in this book. Look for real and perceived similarities between the two of you and bring them up. Mirror their body language, word usage, gestures, and facial expressions. Anticipate their questions and prepare honest answers that will reduce the number of unknowns. All these steps will make the bad news more believable.

Start your conversation with the foundation of what's gone wrong. *State the problem first and then go into details.* Don't string someone along with details first. "Well, Mrs. Smith, as you know, your case started when you noticed the lump in your right breast, so we decided to do a mammogram, and then we decided to do a biopsy, and then we did surgery, and...." Mrs. Smith is thinking, *Oh for crying out loud, just spit it out! Get to the point!* Instead say, "Mrs. Smith, there has been a terrible complication. Here's what happened...." State the problem and then provide the details and clarification.

When you're delivering bad news, always *use professional language* to make straightforward statements that are backed up by facts. Give clear, scientific explanations. Don't say, "I know this totally sucks," or, "This is a major bummer." No, it is not a major bummer. It is a devastating complication. It is a grim outcome. You are discussing the suffering or death of somebody's loved one. Treat this situation with the gravity it deserves.

Don't sugarcoat things. Just as people can usually taste sugar when it's in a recipe, people can also detect it in a conversation. Tell it like it is. Don't try to minimize something that's major. If there is anything positive to report, by all means include that too—but only after you've delivered the bad news. For example, "We had to sacrifice the facial nerve, but the entire tumor was removed and that will make radiation therapy more successful." That's a great example of following bad news with good in a way that is direct, simple, honest, and professional.

If there is bad news to be delivered and you're the most senior person involved, *don't try to delegate* it. The late author and motivational speaker Jim Rohn used to say, "You can't have someone else do your push-ups for you." You can't pass this task off on some other poor soul on your team. Set aside two minutes to do it yourself. But do take an intern or a nursing student along with you. Let them listen and let them learn, because inevitably they will have to communicate bad news at some point in their career. Be a good role model and teacher for them.

It is OK to say you're sorry. Saying you're sorry simply means you care. It is not an admission of guilt. That has been established by malpractice lawsuit precedent. Saying, "I am sorry for your loss" expresses your empathy, and it is emotionally meaningful for the recipient to hear. Or you can say, "I wish I had better news for you, however...." People appreciate when their doctor shows that they care; that they too wish things had turned out differently.

Be sure to *talk directly to the people who are most affected* by the bad news. You wouldn't go to a nephew and ask him to convey to his aunt the sad news that her husband just passed away. Go straight to the most affected person and tell them first. That is the respectful thing to do. If the most affected person is not in the hospital at that time, you can provide a little bit of information to the ones who are there, but make it clear that your primary objective is to speak with the person closest to the patient.

After delivering the unpleasant news, *offer to answer questions.* In a situation like this, you should expect to field a few inquiries. That is a no-brainer. Communication is a chess game, and you'll need to think two or three steps ahead so you can prepare your answers prior to the discussion. Even when time is pressed and you can't sit for an hour with the family to discuss things in depth and help them process their loss, you can say, "I can take a few moments here and answer any questions you may have. What can I answer for you at this time?" If you don't have the answer to a question, say so. Never estimate or speculate about what may have occurred if you don't know what it actually was.

Remember that *all news is subjective.* What may seem like good or neutral news to you may be devastatingly horrible to someone else, and vice versa. It is strictly a matter of opinion. In healthcare we tend to thrive on some of the milestones within our specialties, and we sometimes get overly caught up in them. Don't do it! Here is an example of what I mean: Let's say you're talking with a single, forty-four-year-old female corporate executive. You start out the conversation by saying, "I have great news! You're pregnant!" A pregnancy may seem like great news to you, but it may be the opposite of that in your patient's mind.

The end of life is the same. *End of life* means different things to different people. While it may appear to be a devastating loss, it may be a relief for the patient's family members, especially if it has been a long, drawn-out, agonizing illness. The passing of their loved one may actually be a weight off their shoulders. They may view it as a blessing that their loved one is now pain-free. Deliver all news with a matter-of-fact demeanor. State the truth in a professional manner using details and scientific information, and let the conversation go from there. It usually doesn't take long to get a feel for the situation.

Avoid placing blame or making excuses. Excuses and blame serve no purpose. They provide no solutions to a problem, and they make you look bad. Remember the chapter on spontaneous trait transference? If you don't want the blame to come right back to you like a boomerang, don't trot it out in the first place.

You are the bearer of bad news. Bear it and move on. Blaming someone else doesn't change the factual outcome of what you're conveying, so convey it concisely. I believe it was Franklin Roosevelt who came up with the three B's of public speaking: be sincere, be brief, and be seated. I think that's great advice in medical communication as well.

Lastly—and probably most importantly—*empathize.* This circles back to everything I've written in this book up to now. Put yourself in the other person's shoes. How would you feel if you were in their situation? Treat the patient and their family accordingly. Everybody grieves differently, and I don't mean grieving specifically about a death but about bad news in general. We all grieve when we receive bad news. It is an emotional defense mechanism. Therefore you may witness anger and untoward outbursts when you have to deliver a distressing report. Remain calm and empathize with the fact that they are scared. They have sustained a loss, and they are reacting to that in an emotionally defensive way. It's not necessarily a reflection on you personally. It is a reflection of how they're hurting. This is not the time to get into a yelling match about what they just said. Silence is an excellent weapon of defense in situations like this.

In fact silence is sometimes the best method of communication there is. Sitting silently beside another person in their grief is one of the greatest gifts you can give them. And if you really stop to think about it, there's a pretty special gift in it for you too.

ACTION POINTS

1. *Communicating bad news is a major challenge for most healthcare providers. The basic rules for conveying bad news include:*

   a. *Tell the truth. Deception and half truths are lies and serve no positive purpose in medical care.*

   b. *Reveal it, don't conceal it. You rarely protect anyone by concealing facts. Don't conceal the truth, not even for a short time.*

   c. *Address bad news in a timely manner. You will inevitably be asked, "How long have you known about this?"*

   d. *Establish rapport by mirroring body language, word usage, gestures, and facial expressions.*

   e. *State the problem first, then go into details. Don't string someone along with details; patients or family members may perceive that as avoidance.*

   f. *Use professional, concise language and don't try to minimize major issues.*

   g. *Do not delegate conveying bad news. Speak directly and initially with the people who are most impacted.*

   h. *Answer questions, and remember that bad news – for some – is subjective. Deliver all news with a matter-of-fact demeanor and allow the conversation to evolve.*

Between a Rock and a Hard Place

Who speaks to the instincts speaks to the deepest in mankind,
and finds the readiest response.

— AMOS BRONSON ALCOTT

I must give credit for much of the content of this chapter to David Lieberman, PhD, author of *Get Anyone to Do Anything,* which is in the Recommended Reading list at the end of this book. I encourage you to pick it up because it will help you immensely, especially in dealing with your most stubborn patients. Until then here are some communication skills and techniques you can use to get through to these challenging people.

First, recognize that the fact that a patient is stubborn doesn't mean they are a bad person. It just means that stubbornness is part of their personality type at the time you are talking to them. Try to keep that in mind, and don't take their willfulness personally. Instead of labeling them as stubborn, try thinking of them as persistent, dogged, tenacious, determined, or persevering. Those are all synonyms for *stubborn* but sans the negative associations.

Now, when you come across a particularly *determined* patient, remember the Franklin effect: a person who has done you a favor in the past is more likely to do you a favor in the future. Therefore try to get the patient to do you the favor of agreeing with you about something right off the bat. If they agree with you once—even if it's about something trivial—they will be more likely to agree with you again when it really counts.

For example you could say to the patient, "Mr. Smith, you probably have better things to do today than be here in the doctor's office, but this is what I'd like you to do...." Of course Mr. Smith believes he has better things to do than be there in the doctor's office. He can't help but agree with you on that point. Now he is more likely to listen to your recommendation.

Similarly you can leverage the law of reciprocation, or the law of reciprocal agreement. You can say something like, "Remember when I prescribed your last medication, and you agreed to take it but you told me it wouldn't work? It turns out you were right all along. Well, now I want to try this new medication...." By taking this approach, you remind the patient of a time when they agreed with you, and you make a new suggestion immediately afterward. They'll be more likely to go along with you if they remember they have agreed with you before.

There is another law you can leverage: the law of scarcity. Everybody knows that demand goes up as products become scarce. When people perceive a thing as limited, they want it more, and they want it now. That is true in economics and it is true in a medical environment as well. Therefore, if there is something you want the patient to do but they are resisting it, try placing a small restriction on their doing that very thing. If you want Bob to try a new medication but he is defiant, tell him, "Bob, I don't want you to start this medication for at least a week. You can't start it until next Sunday."

In Bob's mind you have planted a seed of scarcity. Now he cannot wait for Sunday to arrive so he can finally do the thing he was restricted from doing before—the thing he didn't even want to do in the first place: taking his medication.

Another trick for getting a less-than-enthusiastic patient to agree to your recommendations is to get them to relocate physically from point A to point B. When a person decides to dig in their heels about something, they lock themselves into the chair and create a fortress out of their own body. If you're talking with them and making suggestions but nothing is getting through, often you can get those proverbial fortress walls to crumble by getting the patient to move.

You can say, "You know what, Mrs. Smith? Let's discuss this in my office rather than here in this sterile clinic room." That gets the patient to stand up, walk down the hallway, and change their chair. Or, if you don't want to (or can't) switch to another office, try simply walking to the other side of the room you are in. The patient will have to shift in their seat to see you. Just find some way to get the patient to move, because once they have budged *physically*, they will be more likely to budge *mentally*.

Whether you change rooms or not, always give your patients an out. Let's say you make a suggestion and the patient adamantly refuses to go along with it. You make the suggestion again, and they still refuse. If you intend to make that suggestion a third time, you must offer some semblance of additional information. Otherwise the patient will never agree *even if they really want to*. They'll think, *I told him twice already that I didn't want to do this. Now, I know he's probably right…but I'm going to look like a schmuck if I change my mind, because he hasn't given me a solid reason to do so.*

Give your patients some new information that will allow them to say yes to you yet still save face. In a previous chapter, I encouraged you to say the word *because* after you make a recommendation. This would be a great time to apply that technique *because* it gives your patient something to grab on to—something that will allow them to take their heels out of the sand and agree with you at last. Remember, the rationale for your *because* doesn't even have to make sense for it to be effective.

Another interesting technique is to have the challenging patient sit near a mirror or reflective window when you make recommendations to them. People are more agreeable when they can see their own reflections. So if you're going to make an important request of someone, seat them so that if they glance to the side, they can see their own reflection. They will be more likely to go along with your recommendations when they know someone is watching—even if they are that someone.

Yet another helpful technique for swaying an adamant patient is to provide a two-sided argument for them. When you, the requestor, are open enough to state both sides, it makes it easier for the patient to consider both as well. Let me give you an example of this. I want my patient to quit smoking. I can say, "I understand that this is America. If I were you, I would probably think that I can do whatever I want, right? However, doing what you want may not be the best choice in this situation because...."

I provided the patient with both sides of the argument. First I acknowledged her side—that this is America, she has a choice, and she can choose to do whatever she wants. Then I gave her my side. Always give the patient both sides of the argument. By saying, "If I were you, I would probably be thinking..." and then following that with your recommendation, you're rationalizing what you expect them to say, and that tells them you're ahead of them in this conversation. That tells them you have thought about it from all angles and you're making a rational decision based on information from both sides, not just your own opinion. That makes you a more rational debater and a more believable, persuasive person.

And then lastly, let the patient think it was their idea all along. You can say something like, "Mrs. Smith, I suspect you've been thinking about this for a long time," or, "You've been testing me on this, haven't you,? Or my personal favorite, "Obviously you were way ahead me on this one, Mrs. Smith!" Even after the patient has agreed with you, go ahead and throw a comment like that out there. If you do, she will take pride in having ownership in the outcome. And even if you had to practically twist her arm to get her to agree to your recommendation, you'll be able to smile on the inside knowing that you helped a challenging person feel better about herself.

ACTION POINTS

1. *Leverage the use of the Franklin effect, the law of reciprocity, and the law of scarcity when trying to persuade a stubborn patient.*

2. *Get the patient to relocate physically or change positions by moving. This triggers a reset of their disagreement and refusal.*

3. *Allow the patient an out – get them to change their mind by offering new information and using the word* because.

Capitalize on Compliments

I can live for two months on a good compliment.

— MARK TWAIN

As you become a better communicator and consequently a better healthcare provider, you will start to receive many compliments from Raving Patients®. People will appreciate the way you communicate with them and care for them, and they will tell you so. That sounds like a good thing, but the truth is that not everyone feels comfortable being complimented, and not everyone knows how to receive a compliment gracefully. If that description fits you, take heart. You can learn to field compliments in a way that helps both you and the other person feel even better.

First and foremost, accept the compliment with a smile. If a patient stands before you and says, "Dr. Wonderful, you have been just fantastic through all of this," don't respond with, "It's just part of the job." If you say that, you're going to come across as a pompous ass. Of course it's a part of the job. You're not telling them something they don't already know. Instead simply accept the compliment with professionalism and with gratitude. It is perfectly fine to reply to with, "That is very kind of you to say," or, "Words like that just make my day." Those are appropriate responses to a compliment. In so many words, you have thanked them for their thoughtfulness and consideration.

Often you will receive indirect compliments. Acknowledge those appropriately too. I consider referrals from another patient or doctor to be the ultimate compliment. In sending a loved one or a patient your way, they are entrusting that person to your care. Accept that and be grateful for it. Whenever I see a new patient, I always start the conversation by asking, "So, who can I thank for sending you my way?" At the end of that visit, I take thirty seconds to jot a note of gratitude to that referring patient or doctor (with the patient's permission, of course). I want them to know I appreciate their kindness in recommending my services. By doing so I send that compliment—that good energy—back out into the world.

Another indirect compliment occurs when someone says to you, "All the surgery nurses said you were the best." An appropriate response to that would be to reciprocate the compliment by saying, "Wow, that's so nice to hear! They are a fantastic bunch, aren't they? I should buy them some donuts." This response capitalizes on spontaneous trait transference. When you answer an indirect compliment with a sincere compliment of your own, you will be viewed as a nice person.

However, watch your step. Too much of a good thing can be exactly that: too much. Compliments are like Oreos. I love them, but I don't want forty of them shoved down my throat. An overabundance of compliments from a patient can signal a borderline personality disorder, a passive-aggressive type of situation, or the presence of an ulterior motive. If there are too many compliments coming your way, register that in your communication bank. And when compliments start to stack up on top of each other, return the conversation to the medical task at hand. You can say, "That's very kind of you. Now, how can I help you today?" or, "Let's stay focused on how I can help you," or, "Thank you. Now let's talk blood pressure."

Sometimes what starts as a chain of compliments ends up as a sexual innuendo or outright sexual advance by the patient. Believe me, it happens. I suppose you could call that the ultimate compliment, but it is not one we will accept as professional healthcare providers. When that line is crossed, silence is an excellent weapon. Pause and wait silently for a moment. If the patient does not get the message, then it is perfectly fine to put your hand up and say, "Stop now." Maintain eye contact and have a blank expression on your face when you say that. That signals you are serious. You can also say:

- "We will move forward in an appropriate manner or this visit is over," or,
- "Your statements [or actions] now are inappropriate and must stop," or,
- "Everything discussed here will be appropriately documented," or,
- "We've come to the end of our appointment."

Occasionally the patient's behavior is so improper that you have no choice but to dismiss them from your care. Refer to the chapter entitled "Let the Ax Fall on Dead Trees" for instruction on how to do that properly.

ACTION POINTS

1. *Compliments come in all manners and varieties. Accept them with professional grace and a statement of gratitude.*

2. *When receiving a conveyance of a compliment about you made by someone else, reciprocate with a compliment about the originator and activate the law of spontaneous trait transference.*

Criticism: The Gift That Keeps on Giving

*Criticism is something we can avoid easily by saying nothing,
doing nothing, and being nothing.*

— ARISTOTLE

I am sure I don't need to tell the doctors and other seasoned health-care professionals who are reading these pages that criticism runs rampant in the medical field. There's just no way around it. Fortunately the days of swearing at one another, throwing instruments around the operating room, and belittling colleagues at morbidity and mortality conferences have given way to more constructive criticisms delivered in a civil manner. Still, it is never easy to be on the receiving end of criticism, especially when it is delivered in an inept way.

But criticism is actually a good thing. It helps us improve. It gives us new perspectives about the way we're doing things. It gives us humility—and many of us don't have enough of that. It helps us think rationally. It helps us mitigate our constant need to be right. Criticism is how we move from one stage of learning to the next, and it always has been. And eventually, as we make changes based on criticism, it helps our self-confidence and helps us learn to deal with discomfort.

Accepting and utilizing criticism is important not only for improving our future medical decisions but also for improving our lives outside of work. For example surgeons are notorious for not being open to criticism. Unfortunately they are also more likely to take adverse events and other negative experiences home with them, much to their (and their loved ones') detriment. Research proves it. A 2005 study[28] of a group of Norwegian physicians showed there is a negative impact on the personal and family lives of healthcare providers when they feel responsible for an adverse event that harmed a patient, and this is directly correlated with their level of accepting criticism. Participants were asked if they accepted criticism well or were at least open-minded about it. Those who responded "no" were the same people who felt far worse in their personal lives following an adverse event. Therefore, the better you are at accepting criticism and utilizing it, the better you will fare personally and professionally.

There are two types of criticism: constructive and deconstructive. "Dude, you're an ass" is deconstructive criticism. Not helpful. On the other hand, constructive criticism is "I think there is a better way to do this, and I'd like to tell you how." No matter how it's delivered, when it comes to hearing criticism about yourself, you have a choice. You can choose to take it and benefit from it or you can choose not to accept it at all.

There's an old story that illustrates this beautifully. Once upon a time, the Buddha was delivering a lecture when he was suddenly interrupted by a man who leveled a flood of verbal abuse against him. The Buddha waited until the man finished his tirade and then asked, "If a man offered a gift to another but the gift was declined, to whom would that gift belong?"

The man politely responded, "It would belong to the man who offered it to begin with."

---

28 O.G. Aasland, R. Førde, "Impact of feeling responsible for adverse events on doctors' personal and professional lives: the importance of being open to criticism from colleagues,"*Quality & Safety in Health Care* 14, 1 February 2005): 13–7, accessed February 2, 2013, http://www.ncbi.nlm.nih.gov/pubmed/15691998.

The Buddha said, "Then I decline to accept your abuse, and I request that you keep it for yourself."

So consider criticism a gift, and remember that you can choose to accept gifts or you can choose to leave them with the giver. To help yourself make that choice, first consider the source. Empathize with the person who is offering you criticism. Put yourself in their shoes. Imagine what secondary gain they may have in giving that criticism. If they have none, then it is probably an honest critique. It is probably something that is being offered up to help you improve and move forward.

Next, really listen to the criticism and look for a solution within it. Offering criticism without also offering a solution serves no purpose. That is deconstructive. It is negative and designed to break people down. I tell my coworkers that I always want to hear their complaints, but only if those complaints come with solutions attached. If someone complains without offering a solution, then they're just bitching. Don't accept the negative. If somebody tells you, "Dude, you're an ass," that is not a criticism you should accept because there is no solution attached. Focus only on that which is helpful.

Accept criticism with a smile. If you immediately go on the defensive with someone who is offering you criticism, you are breaking down their ability to convey it to you properly. Smile, nod, and listen to what they have to say because at that point you're dealing only with words. It is your choice to accept them or not. Be a grown-up. Communicate calmly, confidently, and quietly in a way that shows you are willing to take your critic's views into consideration. Quiet confidence is like a nuclear weapon in the communication wars. Whether you are facing constructive or deconstructive criticism, it will always be the best weapon in your arsenal.

Respond with gratitude for the person-offering-the-criticism's effort to help you improve. In their mind they are trying to make things better. If they offer no background or solution, respond with, "Tell me why you feel that way," or, "I wish I knew why you would say that." Take it in. Process it, and if a response is merited, keep it positive. Rarely will defensiveness and argumentative responses help a situation improve. If you do not agree, simply say so. "I may not agree with you on that but I honor your opinion" might be a kind effort to find closure to the criticism. If they are right, acknowledge it. You don't have to admit fault, but you can "take it under advisement," as our legal colleagues say. You might respond with, "You know, I can see where you're coming from," or, "I hear what you're saying."

Whether the criticism you receive is complete nonsense or a revolutionary way to improve yourself, you have the choice to accept or decline it. Do so professionally.

ACTION POINTS

1. *Criticism is a gift offered to you by someone else. You have the choice to accept it or decline it.*

2. *Research proves that the better you are at accepting criticism and utilizing it, the better you will fare personally and professionally.*

Kittens and Puppies Are Not
Cats and Dogs

A person's a person, no matter how small.

— Dr. Seuss

Children are not little adults who just happen to process information inefficiently. They are a special genre of patients who happen to think differently than others. Too often healthcare providers walk into the exam room, talk exclusively to the child's parent, then walk out. They treat children like inanimate objects — as furniture. But kids deserve to be treated with respect and communicated with as individual human beings, and I'm going to tell you how to do that effectively. I am going to bypass the baby-toddler stage for obvious reasons and begin with ideas for communicating with children aged three to six.

Let's say you and a preschooler were to pour a jug of water onto a tilted table and then watch together as that water ran down onto the floor. If you were to ask the child, "Why did that happen?" they would have no idea, nor would they care. They would just think it was pretty cool. They'd probably giggle and put their hands in the water. They'd probably stomp in it and make it splash because water is pretty when it sparkles. They wouldn't care why the water ran down the table. They would simply take it for the visual and physical characteristics it presented. They would enjoy it and then move on.

Essentially they're like little Buddhas who exist in the moment all the time. So if one comes to you with an earache and you try and explain to him why his ear hurts or outline the reason why you have to do surgery, you are just wasting everybody's time. It's as if you're trying to explain the effect of gravity on the water running down the table. They are not going to care in the least. To communicate effectively with this subset of patients, you have to communicate with the parents while still keeping the children as the focus. Allow them to be wherever they want to be. Point out things in the room that sparkle or that make funny noises. Hand them your stethoscope. Let them sit on a parent's lap. Let them move around. That's fine. They are existing in their own little world. Let their moment be their moment, and communicate the treatment plan to their parent or guardian.

You can take a different approach with six- to nine-year olds. If you pour the water down the tilted table and ask them why the water fell to the floor, they will manufacture a reason. They will say something like, "Because it wanted to," or, "Because the water fairy made it fall down." Children in this age group like to think there is a reason for everything. The reason doesn't necessarily have to make sense — there just has to be one.

This refers back to the earlier chapter where we discussed the power of the word *because*. People will generally let you cut in line for the copy machine as long as you give them a reason, even if the reason is nonsense. Remember that when communicating with this age group. Six- to nine-year olds want to know that there is a reason they're in your office, so use the word *because* with them. If you tell them they're there *because* they have an ear infection, they'll usually be content with that. You don't necessarily have to spend a great deal of time explaining things to them. Just state the reason on a level they can understand and then continue the conversation with the parent or guardian.

The ten-year-old to adolescent age group can probably tell you exactly why the water is running down the table. Most of them will say it has to do with gravitational pull. The more intellectual children might launch into an explanation of how the surface tension of the water overcomes the friction of the surface of the table, or how the momentum and kinetic energy of the water propel it down the table equivalent to the gravitational pull. There might even be that one kid who points out that if you stand on your head, the water isn't running downhill at all. These are people who try to understand why things happen. These are people you have to talk to directly. Introduce yourself to them first and then address their parent. Let them know they are the important one in this relationship.

Within this age group—especially among those in the adolescent ranks—you will find some who are very tough to communicate with. There are defense mechanisms and walls that adolescents put up to help them cope and exist inside their own little box. Sometimes they are resistant to communication because they don't want to be wrong. They don't want to embarrass themselves. So utilize the power of the Franklin effect. Get them to agree with you and do you a favor right off the bat and they'll be more likely to do you the favor of agreeing with you later on about their treatment.

"I probably remind you of your grandfather," you say, "but I'm going to do my best to help you out." They think, *Yeah, you do remind me of my grandfather...* Or you could say, "Wow, that's a sharp phone you've got there. I doubt I could use it as well as you can." Of course they're thinking exactly the same thing! Now the stage is set for both of you to move forward.

Those are a few of the differences between various age groups. Next let's explore some of the nonverbal communication we can use to make children feel more comfortable.

First, choose an environment that isn't scary, and make the little patient comfortable. If a child comes in to have a mole removed, you can do so in a comfortable room with the child sitting in a recliner just as easily as you can in a sterile, white room with tile floors and a surgical table. I can tell you which one is more relaxing for the child. I've done surgery in both, and children are far more agreeable to what you suggest when they are in a comfy environment. I've stitched up lacerations with a child lying on a parent's shoulder with their head turned. I've stitched up lacerations with little people sitting in their car seats. Wherever they are most comfortable is the best place for them to be. They don't have to be up on a sterile metal table. Truly, do they? You can listen to their lungs when they're sitting on a parent's lap or while they're playing with blocks on the floor. Move to their level. If they're down on the floor, kneel or sit on the floor with them. Sometimes that's what it takes. I have to say, if you are too cool for that then do all of us a favor and get a different job.

Second, smile. Always smile. Children are attracted to smiles like magnets, and they'll likely return them. When you smile at a child, their parent smiles too. The parent needs to know you care for their child. Their main objective in life is to protect their child. If you walk in smiling and introduce yourself in an honest, caring way to their youngster, they will feel more comfortable. It is an honor and a gift when someone allows you to control and even change the most important person in their life. I don't think we doctors and healthcare professionals acknowledge that often enough. Thank that parent for allowing you to take care of their treasured little one.

Third, put the parents at ease. Children are very observant. We don't give them enough credit for that. They will definitely watch how their parents react to you. If you can get the parent to smile and laugh and enjoy meeting you, the child will feel more comfortable and will likely smile and laugh and enjoy meeting you as well. So greet the child and the parents with equal warmth and compassion.

Fourth, always acknowledge what they say. In some cases what they say may be complete and utter nonsense, but you still need to acknowledge it. You need to smile and react to it. If a patient says there's a fairy princess in her ear, it's okay to say, "Wow, there is? Well, let's take a look at her then." You have to acknowledge their belief systems. Children are not just little adults who are mentally ill. They are little patients who think differently.

Fifth, eliminate the unknown. Children fear mystery. They fear what's behind the closet door, and they fear what may be lurking underneath their bed in the dark of night. A doctor's office and all its equipment can be very scary. If you want to hide your equipment behind your young patients and not let them see what's going on, you can, but I don't think it's a very efficient or kind way to move forward in a procedure. I'm on the side of showing them everything. Say, "Look, this is how a stitch is attached to the little needle.... See how this clips into my needle holder? Pretty cool, huh? We put in some numbing medicine so there will be no owies...."

Now they understand what's happening and what all the clicks and noises are about. They don't have to wonder or strain to look behind them. They may not *like* what's happening, but at least they *know* what's happening. That's huge.

Finally, there are many words we use in medicine with adults that are not appropriate to use around children. Keep the words you use positive. For example we sometimes say the word *deformity*. Say "appearance" instead. Don't say you're going to "shoot an X-ray." Say you're going to "take a picture." If you're looking at an X-ray and you say, "This finding right here worries me," the child is going to hear that you're apprehensive. But if you say, "This finding right here makes me wonder," you're saying essentially the same thing but in a positive way.

And for heaven's sake, it is certainly OK to call an injury an "owie" when you're talking to a three-year-old. I promise I won't tell your buddies at the gym.

ACTION POINTS

1. *Know that children are not just miniature, inefficient adults. They are patients who think differently yet thrive on acknowledgement.*

2. *The easiest way to put a child at ease is to put her parents at ease.*

3. *Smile, smile, and smile. Even newborn babies instinctively react positively to smiles.*

4. *Whenever possible, allay fear by eliminating the mystery of the unknown.*

Identifying Sensory Differences

Observe, record, tabulate, communicate. Use your five senses.
Learn to see, learn to hear, learn to feel, learn to smell, and
know that by practice alone you can become expert.

— William Osler

We all rely on our senses for communication — for sorting out the information that comes in and for deciding what information will go back out. This sensory processing takes place every waking moment of every day, but the interesting thing is that each of us does it differently. Understanding and capitalizing upon these differences will improve your communication with your patients, coworkers, family members, and friends.

In his fascinating book called *How to Make People Like You in 90 Seconds or Less* (it's on the Recommended Reading list at the conclusion of this book), author Nicholas Boothman described the sensory processing differences and arranged them into three sensory type categories: auditory, visual, and kinesthetic. Generally speaking each of us fits into one of those categories. It's not that there's anything particularly new about sensory types; it's just that Boothman described it best. What's great about it is that when you can identify a person's sensory type, you can change your communication style to register more effectively with them.

The first sensory type is auditory. Obviously these are the people who process information better when they hear it. Not only do they love to engage in conversation, but they are also typically the first ones to initiate dialogue. They will be the first to introduce new topics into an established conversation. Auditory types have highly developed vocabularies and speech patterns. They are very expressive and eloquent. They have a tendency to move their eyes from side to side when they're talking.

Auditory people lean toward occupations that require the use of words. These are the teachers and the counselors among us. These are the writers and the lawyers. They will say things like, "*Tell me* more," "Wow, that *sounds* familiar," "*I heard* somewhere that we should..." or, "That really *rings a bell* with me." They function within an auditory mindset.

The visual types are people who need to see it before they can believe it. They want to see proof. They want to see the algorithm. If you have a patient who is a visual type, he is going to ask you to show him the X-ray so he can look at the fracture himself. If you're trying to explain something to visual people, they will benefit if you show them pictures or diagrams while you're talking to them. These are the patients who will stare at the monitor in the clinic or in the hospital room because they like to watch the lines go up and down. They will probably ask a lot of questions about what they see.

Visual people talk very quickly. Sometimes they speak in a monotone because their speech moves so rapidly there is no time for inflection. They are usually neatly and fashionably dressed in bright colors, and they like to look at themselves in the mirror. They're usually more fit than average. They tend to have good posture. When they speak, they say things like, "*I see* what you're saying," "I think *we see eye-to-eye* on this," "The future *looks bright*," "*Picture* this," or, "Can you *shed some light* on this for me?"

And then we have the kinesthetic type. These are the people who have to "get a feel" for things. They usually have slower speech and gestures, and a lower voice tone. In fact some of them converse so slowly that the auditory and visual types will want to yell, "Get to the point!" Male kinesthetics often have facial hair. Both men and women like to wear clothes with texture and depth. They enjoy jewelry that has edges and angles.

Kinesthetics have hands-on occupations—they are mechanics, carpenters, plumbers, and builders. Generally speaking (there are exceptions, of course) they are not the most physically fit people. What they see in the mirror is not nearly as important to them as what they think or how they feel on the inside. They're sensitive, laid-back, down-to-earth people.

When you meet a patient, how can you quickly glean insight into their sensory type? You can start by asking questions and listening carefully to their responses. For example let's ask some imaginary patients to describe their headaches in detail, and examine the words they use.

- "This is how I *see* my headaches, Doc. " (visual)
- "I *feel* a deep, burning sensation right here." (kinesthetic)
- "It's like my head is just *screaming* at me." (auditory)

Once you have identified your patient's sensory type, you can tailor your communication style to appeal to their sensibilities. You can say to an auditory person, "So, does that ring a bell?" or, "In a manner of speaking..." or, "Yes, Nurse Theo is a hoot!" With a kinesthetic person, try, "This medicine will have you feeling better inside," "I want you to stay in touch with me," or "We can pull some strings here and come to grips with this problem." *Feelings, grips,* and *pulled strings* are kinesthetic words. That patient is going to be more likely to agree with you and understand what you're saying if you use words that are consistent with their sensory type.

With the visual person, simply say, "Visualize this..." or, "Imagine yourself running upstairs..." or, "Can't you just see yourself playing catch with your kids?" or, "Let me shed some light on this for you..." or, "I really hope we see eye to eye on this." Those are terms a visual person will be able to relate to quite easily.

It takes very little effort to learn and apply these simple concepts. As Nicholas Boothman said, "Developing a knack for detecting sensory preferences means paying close attention to others – and this alone makes you more people-oriented." [29] So take the time to learn these techniques and try them out. If you do, each of your patients, regardless of their sensory type, will come away from your meetings convinced that you are both on the same wavelength. And that will make it all worthwhile, I promise.

ACTION POINTS

1. *Identify the patient as an auditory, a visual, or a kinesthetic. Change your communication style and word choices to register more effectively with them. As Nicholas Boothman said, "Developing a knack for detecting sensory preferences means paying close attention to others – and this alone makes you more people-oriented."* [30]

---

29 Nicholas Boothman, *How to Make People Like You in 90 Seconds or Less* (New York: Workman, 2008), 155

30 Nicholas Boothman, *How to Make People Like You in 90 Seconds or Less* (New York: Workman, 2008), 155

Communi-bation

*Most of the shadows of life are caused by standing
in our own sunshine.*

— Ralph Waldo Emerson

When I told my wife that I intended to title this chapter
"Communi-bation" because it is about communicating with one-
self, she said, "I think you'd better keep that to yourself." Pun
intended...I think. But all kidding aside, self-communication is
a serious matter. The ways people talk to themselves and reflect
upon their own places in the world have a major impact on their
overall success in life. Honestly I don't think we doctors are particularly good at reflection and introspection. We don't do them
often enough, and when we do, we go about it all wrong.

Many of the concepts I've learned about self-communication
come from someone I respect greatly and whom I mentioned in
an earlier chapter — Dan Sullivan, founder of Strategic Coach®
and author extraordinaire. I am going to share some of Dan's
ideas on self-communication here because they have been incredibly valuable to me in my own life and medical practice.

The first concept is to surround yourself and your thoughts
with people, ideas, and mindsets that are more about your future
and less about your past. We doctors and healthcare professionals

across the board are people who usually succeeded greatly when we were younger. We succeeded because we are of above-average intelligence. We passed all the tests and brought home straight A's. We were on all the committees and were leaders in all the clubs. Everyone told us we were smart kids. Everywhere we turned there were accolades and awards. And so over time we started to believe our own good press. That belief became ingrained, and we began to dwell on what we'd heard about ourselves in the past: that we were special, ahead of our class, the cream of the crop. We were the biggest fish in a little pond.

But at some point we moved into a group of peers made up of other cream-of-the-crop people, where we were just like everybody else. We doctors tend to find that hard to accept. We were funneled into the larger system, a top-down pressure cooker, and we became just another gear in the machine. It is only by reflecting on what kind of gear we're going to be and in what way we're going to make that machine run that we can find self-fulfillment. It is only through introspection and honest self-communication that we can come out on the other side with a healthy mindset.

Think of it this way: When we are born, we are given a certain amount of muscle on our bodies. We cannot control how much we get. It is what it is. As we grow older, we exercise because it is fun and we eat because we're hungry, and our bones and muscles grow over time. They become what they become. Then we reach a point in our lives—usually it's around the age of thirty—when that muscle and muscle tone begin to diminish. The people who make an extra effort to continue maintaining that muscle mass and building more are the people who are stronger moving forward. They're leaner, more athletic.

It's that way in your career, family life, and marriage as well. It takes work for you to maintain muscle in those aspects of your life. You have to work out. You have to eat right. You have to spend quality time with your family and partner. When it comes to your medical career, you need to continue to educate yourself. You need to continue to reflect on what you're doing and how that's going to make you stronger in the future—or not. Unfortunately I have watched far too many colleagues not keep up with the exercises it takes to build toward their futures, to build the muscle it takes to march forward. They become jaded. They become cynical. They become mean to others. I have watched veteran doctors say to young, aspiring physicians, "If I had to do it over, I would never do this again." And I always want to ask them, "When did you stop working out? When did you stop striving?" Because that's why they feel so discouraged. It is not the medical profession that is making them feel that way. It is their response (or lack of response) to the challenges we face in this industry.

We all change, and the medical environment changes as well. The same people and thought processes that got you here are in all likelihood not the same people and thought processes that are going to get you where you want to be in the future.

First, you have to decide where you want to go. Where is your ability going to take you in the future? What do you foresee that future being? You have to ask yourself that and honestly reflect upon it, then write it down.

Second, you need to act on it. You need to change. Just as we have to change our exercise regimens and diets as we age, so too do we have to change our thinking and our communication skills. We must strengthen them and make them better because the thinking and the communication skills we've had in the past may not be sufficient to take us forward another twenty years.

It's like in the book of Exodus. The person who originally led the people out of Egypt was not the same person who ended up leading them to the promised land. There were forty years of wandering in between. I think everybody's life is a little bit like that. You need to find the person inside yourself and communicate with that person about where the promised land might be and what direction you're going to take to find it. Because if you continue to wander, you'll continue to remain in the desert of a career you don't like. That is not a comfortable place to be. I see this happen to people across the healthcare profession spectrum. I see it happen to nurses. I see it happen to doctors. I see it happen to the ancillary personnel who struggle with the notion that they are limited — that they have gone as far as they can possibly go.

If this describes you, know that this is not as far as you can go. I encourage you to read the "One Final Word Before You Go" section near the end of this book and then start reflecting on your vision of your ideal future. Write down your goals and then act upon them. Find something you can do every single day to get you one baby step closer to that ideal. Flex your muscles. Do whatever it takes to change and to make yourself a stronger, happier healthcare professional going forward. You deserve that, and so do all the patients who will come to you for help in the future.

ACTION POINTS

1. *The ways people reflect upon their own places in the world has a major impact on their overall success in life.*

2. *Surround yourself and your thoughts with people, ideas, and mindsets that are more about your future and less about your past. Those who brought you to where you are now may not be those who take you where you want to be in the future.*

Action Points Summary

It Pays to be Nice. Literally

1) *Before entering the room to see the patient, stop and take note of his or her name. Use it in your greeting and in conversation with the patient.*

2) *If you find yourself relating to a patient in a negative manner (i.e. using a harsh or impatient tone of voice), pause and take a proverbial step to the side and begin again in a positive manner. Your malpractice claims history may depend on it.*

3) *Don't take yourself too seriously. Your current frustration will pass. Smile and know everything will work out ten minutes before it's too late.*

4) *Remember that when you are with a patient, you are never the most important person in the room. Ever.*

Universal Characteristics of Friendship

5) *Establish similarity through mirroring. Mirror body language, word usage, gestures, and facial expressions to establish perceived similarity.*

6) *If you and your patient have a true similarity, mention it. Use it as a starting point for building trust and patient confidence.*

7) *Anticipate common questions and prepare answers that will put your patients at ease. Cooperate in your patients' care by reducing the unknown for them.*

8) *Choose to provide positive suggestions rather than negative criticism. Illustrate the positive outcomes and benefits of your recommendations.*

Dunbar's Number

9) *Be on the lookout for opportunities to be more positive, empathetic, interested, compassionate, and approachable. Make an effort to join your patient's Dunbar's number.*

10) *Mention and capitalize on a nonmedical similarity you have with the patient.*

11) *If your friend breaks his leg, take him a pan of lasagna.*

Choose Your Perception

12) *Before every patient interaction, choose a positive perception of what you expect to happen with that patient.*

13) *When you are called in at an inconvenient time, leave your negative attitude behind. You just might get paid in full — in cash.*

14) *Even if you are in a less than ideal interaction, remember someone is watching you. Stay positive and act professionally. Your reputation depends on it.*

Comfort and Ease

15) *Position yourself in front of the patient at their eye level. Help them achieve a comfortable body position in order to listen better to your recommendations.*

16) *Acknowledge an uncomfortable situation for the patient with reassurance and gratitude for their cooperation.*

17) Smile more.

The Eyes Have It

18) Structure your consultations to include sufficient time for charting and *for active patient engagement, including eye contact — especially during discussions about diagnoses, findings, and treatments.*

19) During the most vital portions of your discussion about diagnoses, findings, and treatments, make certain to establish eye contact with the patient.

20) Determine the patient's eye color. When you know the color of your patient's eyes, you will know that you have established adequate eye contact.

The Pratfall Effect

21) Don't be afraid to let patients see that you are not perfect. It makes you seem more human and less intimidating.

22) With discretion, acknowledge a small foible as it happens. Research shows this will likely put the patient at ease and make you more likeable.

Set a Great Example

23) Set an example for your patients by demonstrating with your actions what you recommend for them.

24) Communicate your example to your patients. For example discuss your favorite healthy meals, your exercise routine, or how you quit a bad habit. Your recommendations will be much more believable, and your patients will be far more likely to follow them.

25) Interact with your patients in the way you would like your coworkers or employees to interact with your patients.

26) Set an example with your appearance. Dress professionally.

The Accidental Compliment

27) When you notice something positive about the patient (weight loss, hairstyle, handbag, etc.), mention it even if you are mid-sentence. A spontaneous compliment is taken as heartfelt and genuine and helps you engage with the patient.

28) If you say something complimentary about your patient to someone else, allow the patient you are complimenting to over-hear you.

29) When your employee or colleague does something positive, com-pliment them and let other people hear it. Compliments boost confidence and foster teamwork.

Write It Down

30) Track your conversations for positives and write notes about them in front of the patient.

31) Minimize your reaction to disappointing negatives. Writing down a negative comment will make the patient feel as if they are in trouble.

Would Someone Please Get the Phone?

32) Mystery shop at your front desk. Have an anonymous friend call in to ask a few questions, then get their feedback on how it went. Use that feedback to devise ways to improve the telephone experience for your patients.

33) Have an in-service training on telephone etiquette so everyone on staff understands how to handle phone calls.

34) Forego any automated answering machine and have a kind, helpful human answer your phone.

35) *Over-animate and accentuate your conversational style when you are on the phone. You and your staff will sound far more positive and eager to help your patients.*

Acknowledge Frustration

36) *Anticipate what a patient's first complaint or frustration may be and acknowledge it. Rarely will you be wrong.*

37) *Fear is a normal defense mechanism for patients. Confirm that for them.*

38) *Know that every day will not go as planned. Accept it. Acknowledge when things are not going well and turn your mind toward positive solutions.*

Hello, Old Friend!

39) *Greet patients you have known for some time the way you would an old friend.*

40) *Remember that the only way to make a friend is to be one.*

My Patient, the Computer

41) *Before making a request of or a recommendation to a patient, provide clear, concise information.*

42) *Just because certain words and terms are clear to you, that does not mean they are clear to the patient. Anticipate the level of understanding of the computer — your patient — before inputting data.*

I've Got a Name

43) *A 2009 study published in the BMJ found that the vast majority of patients under the age of sixty-five said they either don't mind or prefer that their doctors call them by their first names.*

44) *Seize every opportunity to include the patient's name in the sentence when conveying information or making recommendations.*

45) *Try introducing yourself by your name and not your occupation.*

46) *When introducing or discussing coworkers, use their names first and foremost, thereby conveying that the people are more important to you than their job titles.*

The Boomerang Effect

47) *When given the opportunity to gossip to or with a patient, don't. Change the subject with positive comments and compliments.*

48) *Remember: research confirms that speaking negatively about another person casts the speaker in a negative light!*

The Reciprocity Rule

49) *Activate the reciprocity rule with patients first by giving them something of value. This may be an informational brochure, a glass of water, a piece of candy, or even a smile and a compliment.*

50) *When making a recommendation you want the patient to follow, use the patient's name, provide the patient with tangible or intangible value, confirm to the patient that you have provided value, and establish a timeframe (to create a sense of urgency) for following that recommendation.*

Something to Smile About

51) *The act of smiling raises human blood levels of serotonin and dopamine and is therapeutic to patients who smile in natural response to your smile.*

52) *You can activate the reciprocity rule by the simple act of giving smiles to your patients.*

53) *Smile more often and you will feel better more often.*

Emotional Predictions

54) *Before you begin a dialogue with a patient, put yourself in their shoes and predict how they may be feeling. Communicate and acknowledge your empathy in a way that shows the patient you care.*

55) *When you need to end the conversation and interaction with the unending-talker patient, deliver your exit statement directly after an emotional prediction or emotional acknowledgement.*

Body Language

56) *Enter each room with the body language of a person who is meant to be there to make a positive difference in someone else's life.*

57) *Point your belly button (not just your head) at the person to whom you are speaking.*

58) *Use your hands for emphasis and for anchoring important points in your conversation. You can do this with fingers steepled together. Remember the namaste greeting of honor and use a kind nod or steepled hands to convey that you understand.*

59) *Use nods of the head to acknowledge positives from your patient. Nod upward: start with your head in the neutral position and nod up and back to neutral, conveying uplifting confirmation of what the patient said.*

60) *Mirror your patient's body position during a conversation to establish a subconscious connection with them.*

Healing Vocabulary

61) *Cleanse your vocabulary of confidence-killing words like* try, hope *and* but. *Instead use assertive words that command action* (can, will, expect, now).

62) *The word* but *often negates the meaning of the words or thoughts that come before it in the sentence. End your statement where*

you would have previously used the word but *and note the positive effect and power it has on the meaning you want to convey.*

63) *Utilize power words such as* absolutely, certainly, definitely, will, *and* can *to instill confidence in the patient about your recommendations.*

The Franklin Effect

64) *Utilize the Franklin effect by first asking your patient to do you a very small favor. After obliging your first simple request, they will be more likely to honor and follow through on your larger, more meaningful recommendations in the future.*

Anchoring

65) *Start each patient interaction with a mental anchor of positive improvement and the expectation of educating the patient about how they can and will improve.*

66) *Set your own anchor point with the patient within the first ten seconds of your visit by exuding a positive, welcoming demeanor.*

The Three Hundred Rule

67) *Even though you may have had the same conversation and made the same recommendations three hundred times, say it with passion and enthusiasm, as if it were the first time. It may be the first time the patient has ever heard it.*

Practice Unselfishness

68) *Donate your time, money, and/or knowledge anonymously.*

69) *Help where help is needed most, not where you gain the most personal notoriety.*

Get Used To Being Uncomfortable

70) Anticipate and accept that as a healthcare provider, you will be in uncomfortable situations at times. Keep your discomfort to yourself and provide comfort to the patient.

Attitude of Gratitude

71) Each day, take note of what you are grateful for. Write it down or tell someone else.

72) Express your appreciation and say "thank you" to your patients. They are giving you the gift of trust. They are also paying your salary.

73) Show your gratitude to your team members with praise for a job well done.

You've Got the Touch

74) When seeking compliance with your recommendations, consider using an inconspicuous touch on the patient's upper arm.

Pessimism Is a Treatable Disease

75) Pessimism is a disease state and it makes people sick. Recognize it. Is it realism or pessimism?

76) Seek out the reason for pessimism (in your patient or yourself) and put it into the perspective of that for which you deserve to be grateful.

77) If you don't like a situation, take action to change it. If you have no control over the situation, then accept it and move on.

78) In the words of a ten-year-old girl, "Life's too short to be a poop head."

The Lake Wobegon Effect

79) *The Lake Wobegon effect is the natural human tendency to over-estimate our abilities. It occurs in both patients and healthcare providers. Be mindful of it.*

80) *Bear in mind that patients will overestimate the likelihood of their compliance with recommendations. Recommend accordingly.*

81) *Avoid the Lake Wobegon effect by not trying to explain something you know nothing about. Confirm to your patients your wish to know more and then do your research or refer accordingly.*

Gossip Is Not Communication

82) *Remember your obligation to the Health Information Portability and Accountability Act and do not participate in gossip.*

83) *Steer the conversation toward positive circumstances and patient care. Saying bad things about someone else is never helpful.*

84) *There is nothing funny about prejudice. If what the patient is saying is demeaning to or judgmental of another person based on race, sexuality, religion, nationality, or disability, do not participate, and redirect immediately.*

Because. Now. Imagine.

85) *Inserting the word* because *after your recommendation and before the reason (any reason) will greatly increase compliance with your recommendation.*

86) *Use the word* now *when you want your patients to take prompt action on a recommendation. It is a known motivator and adds a sense of urgency.*

87) *Ask your patient to* imagine *a positive result of your recommendations. Doing so plants a positive image in the patient's mind.*

Embedded Commands and Metaphors

88) Use embedded commands within your recommendations to increase patient compliance. (A) Know what you want to convey. (B) Wrap the point with positive words and phrases. (C) Accentuate your embedded commands with a physical marker for emphasis. (D) Practice using embedded commands.

89) Use easily visualized metaphors whenever possible to illustrate your recommendations and the reasons for making them more clearly.

Celebrate Uniqueness

90) Ask open-ended questions to discover something unique about your patient. Celebrating a patient's uniqueness is rapport building at its finest.

91) Make your work environment distinctive and interesting. A unique office is full of smiles, interesting décor, and a fresh way of greeting patients.

92) Thorndike's law of effect means that pleasant experiences are more likely to be repeated; unpleasant ones are not. If you want patients to return, honor your recommendations, and provide referrals, then make their visits with you pleasant experiences.

Medical Office Feng Shui

93) You are not the only one communicating with your patients and staff every day. Your office and its appearance communicate to your patients as well. Your office is an extension of the care you offer to your patients.

94) Have someone you trust tell you the truth — have them "mystery shop" your office and report back to you what your office environment is saying.

95) Consider earth-toned colors, live plants, water elements, and instrumental music to put patients at ease while in your office.

96) Eliminate sign-in sheets and multiuse forms that disclose patients' names to others. Be mindful of files and computer screens that may be visible to other patients.

Traction Control

97) When we are trying to make a point or get through to someone, sometimes we push too hard and become aggressive. When you notice this occurring, pull back, slow down, and allow yourself to regain traction in the conversation.

98) Empathize with the patient and verbally acknowledge his or her frustration.

99) Ask permission to make a suggestion or recommendations when the patient seems frustrated. This gives the patient a new sense of control.

100) Exude gratitude by thanking your patients and your coworkers.

How Old Is Your Patient?

101) Recognize that Matures, Boomers, Generation Xers, and New Millennials benefit from different means and techniques of communication.

102) For Matures, lay out a well-ordered, step-by-step outline of their treatment plan and the outcomes you expect to achieve.

103) For Boomers, present options and then make recommendations. Acknowledge their discomfort and mention the years you have invested in learning how to help them.

104) For Generation Xers, acknowledge that medical care is about managing transitions in one's health.

105) *For New Millennials, highlight the intangible prosperity your recommendations will bring. Communicate with technology whenever you can.*

Rules for Discussing Religion and Politics with Patients

106) *Discussing religion and politics with patients is not recommended.*

Let the Ax Fall on Dead Trees

107) *If you must release a patient from your care, do it yourself in a face-to-face meeting, and document accordingly. Do not release a patient in the midst of an acute or urgent medical care situation. Make sure the patient has access to other medical providers. Give a list of providers to the patient. Follow up with a letter reiterating what was discussed in your face-to-face meeting and enclose a copy of the original provider list.*

108) *Document, document, document.*

Communicating Bad News

109) *When communicating bad news, always tell the truth. Address bad news in a timely manner. Establish rapport by mirroring body language, word usage, gestures, and facial expressions. State the problem first and then go into details. Use professional, concise language and don't try to minimize major issues. Do not delegate conveying bad news. Speak directly and initially with the persons who are most impacted.*

110) *Remember that bad news is subjective. Deliver all news with a matter-of-fact demeanor and allow the conversation to evolve.*

Between a Rock and a Hard Place

111) *Leverage the use of the Franklin effect, the law of reciprocity, and the law of scarcity when trying to persuade a stubborn patient.*

112) *Get the patient to physically relocate or otherwise change their position. This triggers a reset of their disagreement and refusal.*

113) *Allow the patient an out to change their mind by offering new information and using the word* because.

Capitalize on Compliments

114) *Accept compliments with professional grace and a statement of gratitude.*

115) *When receiving a conveyance of a compliment about you made by someone else, reciprocate with a compliment about the originator and activate the law of spontaneous trait transference.*

Criticism: The Gift That Keeps on Giving

116) *Criticism is a gift offered to you by someone else. You have the choice to accept it or decline it.*

117) *Research proves the better you are at accepting criticism and utilizing it, the better you will fare personally and professionally.*

Kittens and Puppies Are Not Cats and Dogs

118) *Know that children are not just miniature, inefficient adults. They are patients who think differently yet thrive on acknowledgement.*

119) *The easiest way to put a child at ease is to put her parents at ease.*

120) *Smile, smile, and smile. Even newborn babies instinctively react positively to smiles.*

121) Whenever possible allay fear by eliminating the mystery of the unknown.

Identifying Sensory Differences

122) Identify the patient as an auditory, a visual, or a kinesthetic. Change your communication style and word choices to register more effectively with them.

Communi-bation

123) The ways people reflect upon their own places in the world have a major impact on their overall success in life.

124) Surround yourself and your thoughts with people, ideas, and mindsets that are more about your future and less about your past. Those who brought you to where you are now may not be those who take you where you want to be in the future.

Recommended Reading

Unstoppable Confidence: How to Use the Power of NLP to Be More Dynamic and Successful by Kent Sayre

How to Make People Like You in 90 Seconds or Less by Nicholas Boothman

Influence: The Psychology of Persuasion by Robert B. Cialdini, PhD

How to Talk to Anyone: 92 Little Tricks for Big Success in Relationships by Leil Lowndes

How to Instantly Connect with Anyone: 96 All New Little Tricks for Big Success in Relationships by Leil Lowndes

Get Anyone to Do Anything by David J. Lieberman, PhD

59 Seconds: Think a Little, Change a Lot by Richard Wiseman

Words That Sell by Richard Bayan

The 80/20 Principle: The Secret of Achieving More with Less by Richard Koch (no relation)

Secrets of Closing the Sale by Zig Ziglar

Getting Everything You Can Out of All You've Got by Jay Abraham

How Successful People Think: Change Your Thinking, Change Your Life by John C. Maxell

Just Listen: Discover the Secret to Getting Through to Absolutely Anyone by Mark Goulston

Motivating the "What's In It For Me" Workforce: Manage Across the Generational Divide and Increase Profits by Cam Marston

One Final Word Before You Go...

Look at today's date on the calendar. Today is the last time you will ever see that day! It will never come again. Every day is like that. You won't get another yesterday. Being happy is a choice that is yours to make! We all have troubles and frustrations. Sorry to break it to you, but you'll have a few more. So what! Quit whining and start making today and tomorrow and the next day awesome. Open your eyes and change the way you see things. Compliment more people. Take more chances. Turn up the music. Get laughed at. State your opinion. Make a mistake (or three). They won't matter a year from now. You get one ticket to this carnival we call life. Ride every ride, eat some cotton candy and try to win a bear. Just go for it! Stop complaining about stuff that doesn't matter and say "Wow! That is really cool!" about stuff that actually does. Prove to yourself you are better today than you were yesterday and announce to anyone who will listen what you will do tomorrow. Our biggest regrets are almost always what we did not do, what we should have tried, what we could have been. Stop regretting! Dump your attitudes and excuses in a place where you put things you don't need anymore. Here's your "carnival" ticket! The turnstile is waiting.

Brent Koch

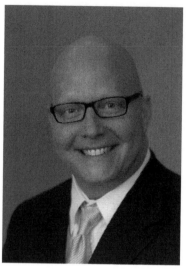Brenton Koch, MD, FACS, is a board-certified facial plastic and reconstructive surgeon, and author of *50 Questions (You MUST Ask!) Before You Have Plastic Surgery.* He is certified by both the American Board of Facial Plastic and Reconstructive Surgery and the American Board of Otolaryngology—Head and Neck Surgery. At his practice in Des Moines, Iowa, plastic surgery of the face is his exclusive specialty. Dr. Koch is supported by administrative and operating-room staffs that are specifically trained to care for plastic and reconstructive surgery patients. Each year his team of professionals prepares for and performs hundreds of facial surgeries treating conditions relating to appearance, accident, or disease.

Dr. Koch completed his undergraduate and premedical training at Drake University in Des Moines. He graduated from the University of Iowa College of Medicine, where he received numerous honors including the Hancher-Finkbine Medallion for outstanding academic leadership contributions to the college. He also earned the American Medical Association National Leadership Achievement Award, which is presented to only twenty recipients nationally.

Dr. Koch completed his residency at the prestigious University of Iowa Department of Otolaryngology—Head and Neck Surgery, which consistently ranks as one of the top programs in the country. He subsequently completed advanced fellowship training in facial plastic and reconstructive surgery at Indiana University and the Meridian Plastic Surgery Center in Indianapolis through the American Academy of Facial Plastic and Reconstructive Surgery. He served as a clinical instructor of facial plastic surgery at Indiana University and is currently a clinical assistant professor of facial plastic surgery with the University of Iowa Department of Otolaryngology—Head and Neck Surgery. He has continued to maintain active involvement in clinical research with numerous publications, research awards, and national presentations to his credit.

Dr. Koch and his wife—Heidi M. Koch, MD, an age-management and functional medicine physician—reside in Des Moines with their four children: Nicole, Blake, Tatum, and Piper. Dr. Koch enjoys sports of all kinds, and as a former college football player, former Ironman, and competitive bodybuilder, he avidly enjoys exercise. His favorite activities, however, are those done with his family.

Dr. Koch is the founder of a charitable nonprofit for underprivileged student athletes called Empower to Play and an enthusiastic supporter of charitable organizations in his community such as the Animal Rescue League of Iowa, Juvenile Diabetes Research Foundation (JDRF), Mercy Medical Center's Mammogram Assistance Fund, and countless other events and causes through donations of his time and services.

Dr. Koch is available for speaking engagements, consulting, and educational forums. While he is an expert in facial plastic and reconstructive surgery and continues in private practice, he has founded a number of healthcare companies including Koch Center for Integrative Health and Spas de Cor, LLC. He has authored three books on various healthcare best practices and is a Clinical Assistant Professor with the University of Iowa Department of Otolaryngology-Head and Neck Surgery continuing to teach medical students and residents personally. Dr. Koch is passionate about and has great insight into healthcare provider communication, internal corporate marketing, private practice development, and making healthcare an exciting, efficient and profitable business. He is an energetic, charismatic speaker and brings a wealth of experience to each engagement whether to large groups in corporate healthcare or individual practices. To schedule an appearance, please email koch@kochmd.com or call 515-277-5555.

Made in the USA
San Bernardino, CA
27 September 2013